OKAY,
SO I DON'T
HAVE A HEADACHE

Also by the author

Cristina Ferrare's Family Entertaining
Cristina Ferrare Style

Cristina Ferrare

OKAY,
SO I DON'T
HAVE A HEADACHE

St. Martin's Griffin ⚜ New York

This book is not intended to be a substitute for professional medical advice. The reader should regularly consult a physician regarding any matter concerning her health, especially in regard to any symptoms that might require diagnosis or medical attention.

Designed by Stanley S. Drate / Folio Graphics Co. Inc.

Library of Congress Cataloging-in-Publication Data

Ferrare, Christina.
    Okay, so I don't have a headache / Christina Ferrare.
        p.   cm.
    Includes bibliographical references.
    ISBN 1-58238-029-5 (hc)
    ISBN 0-312-26366-X (pbk)
    1. Menopause Popular works.   2. Menopause—
Complications—Diet therapy Recipes.   3. Middle aged women—
Health and hygiene Popular works.   I. Title.
RG186.F47   1999
618.1'75—dc21   99-25275
                                                                          CIP

First St. Martin's Griffin Edition: May 2000

10 9 8 7 6 5 4 3 2 1

To Tony, my husband. Many times people have come up to him and said, "How can you let your wife talk in such intimate detail about your sex life?" He never saw it as an embarrassment. He looked at it from the point of view that what we went through should be shared so that both women and men can benefit. What a saint! I'm so grateful, now that the smoke has cleared, that we're still standing, or should I say lying down! I love you.

Acknowledgments

Thanks to God, always to God.

Thanks to Jan Miller for her constant encouragement and belief in me. Her generosity of spirit and gift of friendship leave me speechless at times. She's a true woman's woman. How fortunate I am to have her in my life.

Thanks to Dr. Judith Reichman. You can speak frankly with Dr. Reichman and know you will receive an open, honest answer. She makes you feel safe. If it weren't for her, I probably would not have had the nerve to move forward with this project. I value her opinion and her input. Thanks, Judith! Oh, happy day when I finally found you!

Thanks to my friends at Golden Books, Bob Asahina, Cassie Jones, and Ellen Jacob.

Thanks to women everywhere. I love how special we are! We share something wonderful together: our womanhood.

Contents

Bibliography

OKAY,
SO I DON'T
HAVE A HEADACHE

Foreword

The information in this book has been gathered from my own caregivers, other medical experts, and authoritative sources, but the book contains no preferred or endorsed medical point of view. I can only describe the results I have experienced from the methods I learned on my own. The health benefits and/or risks for you depend on your own personal health profile. Every person is unique. What works for one individual may not work for another.

The herbal and vitamin regimen I suggest in this book comes from a specialist in herbal medicine with whom I have spent long hours to determine the benefits I would receive. This regimen is specific to my individual needs.

You should consult your own caregivers before starting any individual treatment, diet, or exercise regimen. If you are not satisfied with your results, try other regimens until you are.

1

Hitting a Nerve

D id you have any idea your remarks would hit such a nerve?" Oprah asked me. Oprah! How did I end up in Chicago with Oprah Winfrey asking me about my sex life? It was all so surreal. I felt as if I had gone through the looking glass. There I was on national television, telling I don't know how many millions of people that I no longer had a sex drive. I had for so long admired this extraordinary person, and here she was, questioning me about a very intimate part of my life. Of course I told her everything.

How did my one little remark on my own talk show, *Home and Family,* lead to this? Evidently I did hit a nerve with a lot of people; their reactions left me completely stunned.

This is just one of the hundreds of letters I received:

> *I can't tell you how many times I have cried myself to sleep over my inability to enjoy my sexual relationship with my husband. I, too, have a husband who has been very loving and patient. There have been many nights that he thought he wasn't doing something right . . . but it just wasn't the case. It was me, and I didn't know why. I am thirty-eight years old.*
>
> *I spoke to my thyroid doctor about this, but he brushed me off. I do know that his nurse took down my complaints and said, "Oh, your libido is down," and that was that! I have been too embarrassed to speak to my ob/gyn about this (also a male doctor). I have now been off all medications for a year and a half and continue to accept the sentence that I have been given. I am now trying to get up enough courage to make an appointment with my obstetrician to discuss my problem with him. I'm so embarrassed!*
>
> —Rachel, California

It all started when Dr. Andrew Weil appeared as a guest on *Home and Family*. He had written the best-selling book *Eight Weeks to Optimum Health*, and we were doing a segment on women's health issues. He mentioned that women who were in perimenopause, the time before menopause, often suffered from a lack of sexual desire.

"Oh my god, that's me!" Did I say it just in my head? Oh, no, not I. I grabbed Dr. Weil's arm as if he were saving me from drowning and said out loud—really loud—"That's me!" Everyone on the set was absolutely dumbfounded. I quickly added that I enjoyed sex with my husband once we got going, but it took me a little longer to get jump-started these days. Once I did, I was thoroughly in the moment—I was perfectly content just to lie in my husband's arms until I died.

Yes, I, Cristina Ferrare—wife, mother, stepmother, grandmother, daughter, sister, ex-model, actress, chef, author, talk show host—had lost interest in sex. Could it be that I was just tired? How could what was once the most exciting, passionate, and best thing on earth no longer be on my list of must-haves?

It certainly had nothing to do with my husband, Tony. I am insane for the man. We had always enjoyed each other with uninhibited sexual lust. What in the world was going on here?

I have a husband whose sexual appetite frankly puzzles me. He gets up at 5:30 A.M. and runs five miles. Then he gets ready for the office and helps send our girls, Alexandra, twelve, and Arianna, nine, off to school. He goes to one of the many meetings he will have during the day and works at full speed until he gets home at seven or eight o'clock, then he plays with the kids and double-checks their homework (as if I don't know how to!). If it's a night for a business dinner, he showers and we run off, with me usually dragging behind. We get home around 11:30, and then he wants to jump on me. Doesn't he want to sleep?

After my outburst, Dr. Weil simply looked at me and said in a very matter-of-fact tone, "You should have your testosterone checked." Testosterone? Isn't that a guy thing? He went on to explain that women indeed have testosterone, and that it plays an extremely important role in their libido. He said that a very low count or no count would probably turn out to be one of the reasons that I had no sexual desire.

I had noticed my problem about a year earlier and simply accepted that that's the way I was going to feel for the rest of my life. But here was Dr. Weil telling me that a simple blood test would tell the tale. Great, I thought, I'll get some testosterone—whatever that is—use it, and I'll be back! (Not that simple, I later found out.) I made the decision right then and there that I was going to do something about this. I was too young to live the rest of my life without wanting sex. Plus, I was married to a man who wanted to have sex a lot.

The first thing I did was to look for a woman doctor. I have seen male doctors all my life, and they can be incredible. But with all due respect to male physicians, for this problem I wanted to find a woman doctor, someone who had been through pregnancies, PMS, swollen breasts, water retention, and perimenopausal symptoms. I wanted someone who understood that when I told her I wanted to kill the kids, I didn't really need a psychologist.

I contacted Dr. Judith Reichman, who happened to appear on *Home and Family* the week after Dr. Weil, to talk about her new book, *I'm Too Young to Be Old.* I read it from cover to cover and found it to be very helpful. A lot of the things she wrote about made sense to me.

One chapter that caught my eye was on natural hormonal treatment and how hormones affect everything in your body. I knew in my gut that this was the answer I was looking for.

I had already made the decision that I did not want to take synthetic hormones; the natural way was something I wanted to explore. I wasn't content to go to my doctor's office and have him tell me it was time to go on hormone replacement therapy, hand me a package, and say, "Call me in the morning if you feel funny." I knew that in order to make an educated choice I needed to find out about all the alternatives.

I went to the bookstore and bought everything I could on natural hormone replacement. The more I read, the more I realized that not only are there many different ways to replace hormones, but what you eat plays an extremely important role in how your body reacts. I will discuss this later in the book.

Dr. Reichman gave me a complete physical. After the usual routine, she had some blood drawn to determine my testosterone level. The results came back: I had none! She prescribed a 2 percent testosterone cream that I was to apply vaginally two or three times a week.

When I used it for the first time, I instantaneously felt a warm, tingly sensation. The cream also acts as a lubricant if you have any vaginal dryness. It got results for me rather quickly, which Dr. Reichman said is unusual. Lucky me!

I must caution you, the cream is not a miracle. So many women have gone into Dr. Reichman's office asking for the cream as if it were The Cure. Rather, it may be part of the solution to getting your libido on track. I was very fortunate that the cream worked for me, but I also made some changes in my diet that increased the amount of estrogen in my body. Although I would sometimes fall back into my old patterns of eating, I kept at it and developed some delicious new recipes, which I provide later in this book. I am convinced that this problem is solvable—I used myself as a guinea pig!

Of course, I couldn't wait to share the news with my *Home and Family* audience. During our show, my cohost, Michael Burger, and I talked about things that were happening in our lives. Since everyone already knew what was going on in mine, I mentioned what a find this cream was. Boy, did I open up a Pandora's box. The following week I was horrified to find out that I was in one of the tabloids, with the headline screaming, "Ex-supermodel Cristina Ferrare

Loses Her Sex Drive!" So much for speaking my mind on national television.

But from that one article came an interesting phone call. Someone from *Dateline NBC* called to ask if I would be willing to speak to their correspondent Dr. Bob Arnot. He was doing a piece on women and testosterone, and would I be interested in talking to him about the testosterone cream I was using? I agreed to do the interview because I knew there was no one else out there talking to women about what happens when you start to go through menopause, other than night sweats, lack of menstruation, and perhaps starting on hormone therapy. To my knowledge, no one had mentioned that it was possible that you would lose your desire for sex. I wanted to talk about what had happened to me, because I knew I couldn't be the only one who felt this way, although for many long months I thought I was, and was too ashamed to admit it.

I wasn't about to go quietly into "the change." I wanted answers, and I knew I would get feedback from the *Dateline NBC* piece. But I was simply floored by the amount of E-mail I received. What surprised me the most was that the majority of women who wrote to me were between twenty-four and thirty-eight years old. Here I was ready to help my fellow Baby Boomers get through this transition when I realized that this was a larger, more serious problem than I thought, involving women of all ages.

I was really surprised by the next turn of events.

My assistant said to me, "Oprah's show is on the line, and they would like to know if you would come to Chicago and discuss your lack of sexual desire and that cream you're using."

"Are you serious?" I said, not believing my ears. "*The* Oprah wants me to be on her show? Why?"

The *Oprah* producers had done a focus group to find out if this subject was interesting to people. Evidently it was—so many people were desperate to find some answers, or just wanted to know that others were going through the same problem. The producers contacted Dr. Reichman as well, so they could have an expert medical opinion. Who could be more perfect, since she was the one who prescribed the cream to me in the first place?

Next thing I knew, I was heading to Chicago. As I mentioned before, it was truly like going through the looking glass. How many afternoons had I sat and enjoyed watching Oprah's show? After more than ten years on the air, she really seems like someone you know, and her studio becomes an extension of your own living room. And there I was, on the other side. Before I even knew it, I was sitting in one of those big, cushy chairs right next to her. Her presence puts you at ease immediately.

In the front row were eight couples who had similar tales to tell. The women were all very much in love with their mates, but were devastated that their desire for sex was completely gone. They shared their stories, and I began to feel a sense of relief myself when I realized I wasn't wrong in pursuing this. My heart went out to everyone, especially the husbands or mates, who were very loving and supportive, but also perplexed and worried about the whole thing.

This, I'm sure, is when problems start in a relationship. Resentment can build on both sides. The man feels that maybe it's his fault—that he is no longer desirable to his mate. The woman starts to feel guilty, and may even start a fight just to get out of "doing it." Been there!

I used every excuse in the book. *I have a headache* (my favorite). *I have my period, and I'm hemorrhaging. I'm too stressed out from the day, and my back is in a spasm. The car wouldn't start. My nails are wet* (even though I had a manicure the day before). *I cut myself shaving my leg, and I have to keep it elevated.* The list goes on and on. Sometimes I would even go to bed later, hoping he would be asleep by the time I crawled in next to him. (That never worked very well—I swear the man has radar.)

After we finished taping the show, Dr. Reichman and I were asked to stay and continue our conversation with the audience. There were still so many questions to be answered that Oprah wanted to keep on talking while they kept taping. The one big question of the day was from Oprah: "Girl, where do you get the cream?"

After the show aired, I couldn't go anywhere without people stopping me. On the street, in the grocery store, at the flower market—in the carpool lane, for heaven's sake!—women told me about their situations and asked where, oh, where to find the cream. That's when I knew I needed to write a book. I started out meaning to write only about my own experiences, but since I heard from so many people across the country, I wanted to include some of their concerns. Maybe you can recognize yourself in some of these letters. I sure did.

As I listened to your story, I began to cry because I have been experiencing the same problem. I am thirty-one years old, so I know it isn't connected to menopause. I realize that whatever is happening to me is not my fault, and I am going to talk to my doctor about it. Thank you so much for sharing this and making me and others realize it's not our fault!

—Lisa, New Hampshire

I have been so ashamed for so many years about my lack of libido. I'm only thirty-seven, married to a wonderful man for thirteen years, and have two boys. I thought I was a freak. I've never mentioned this to anyone! Well, once to a doctor, who just blew it off. Just recently (this past Monday, in fact) I did mention to my best friend that I finally have a sex drive again!

I honestly believe these newly refound feelings came as a result of weaning myself off Prozac during the holidays (how brave am I?) and switching to St. John's Wort (of course, my doctor isn't happy with the switch to an alternative treatment). It's been during this transition that I've finally started feeling like a real wife/woman—I actually want "it." (And my husband's loving it!)

It's been so awful thinking that I was all alone in this. . . . As with my fibromyalgia and depression, I wouldn't wish this on anyone, but it was comforting to find that I wasn't alone.

—Kathy, Ohio

I'm in my thirties, my mother is in her fifties, and my grandmother is in her seventies. We all watched you on Oprah yesterday and couldn't believe our ears! You were describing us! None of us is on medication. We are just in need of some explanation for our feelings (or lack of!). It would be great if you could give some more information about food and how some foods are better for estrogens. We would really like to try that route.

—Erica, Maryland

Your persistence in seeking a solution to your problem is commendable as well as an example for millions of women out there who are suffering from the same thing. Next to the birth of a child, a healthy sex life, under the covenant of marriage, is a wonderful and beautiful thing. Thanks again for sharing your experience with others.

—Mary Ellen, Michigan

2

I'm Not a Doctor, I Just Play One on TV

I've been hosting talk shows for almost fifteen years. I started in Los Angeles hosting *A.M. Los Angeles*. Since then I've hosted many different talk shows: *The Home Show, Good Morning America,* a series of specials called *Shame on You,* my own shows, *Cristina and Friends, Home and Family,* and others too numerous to mention.

During my career I've met everyone who is anyone. Guests would stop by whatever show I was hosting to promote their latest movie, television show, or book. I've learned so much over the years and put it to use in my everyday life.

I can change the oil in your car—and actually cook a meal on the manifold. (I'm not kidding—I learned that on *Home and Family.*) I've found out when to start perennials, what perennials *are*. I've learned how to reupholster a chair for ten dollars. I'm always up on the latest best-seller or the newest innovations in breast cancer surgery and mammography. I actually had a mammogram on the air so I could show women that it doesn't really hurt. I was okay until we had to go to commercial and the power went down. Then they couldn't release the machine right away. There is something to be said about your breast being flattened, looking like a fried egg as you look down through the Plexiglas. Not fun!

I've covered it all. God only knows, I have an opinion on *everything!* I love my job. I've traveled to wonderful, exotic locations and met some of the world's most interesting people. Still, it always surprises me when I go to an industry function in town and someone important says, "Well, hello, Cristina, how are you?" For some reason I think that no one ever remembers my name, or me.

One of the things I loved best was to substitute host for *Regis and Kathie Lee.* I first did it when Kathie was on maternity leave with her second child, Cassidy. I became the regular sub when Joy, Regis's fabulous wife, was not available. I swear I used to hope Kathie would catch a cold! Not a bad one, just enough for her to decide she needed to stay home. I just loved doing that show! I was always nervous because Kathie is so loved by her audience, and I was aware that I was sitting in someone else's chair, but the exposure I got was invaluable and I will always be grateful to Regis for being so gracious and generous. He is a gem. Working with him was definitely a dream come true for me.

On my own show, the one thing I have always believed in, and try to do on every segment, is leave the audience with one bit of information that they didn't know before. I've always been particularly interested whenever we had a medical segment, especially on nutrition and alternative medicine. I usually keep right on asking questions during commercial breaks. I store a lot of information in my head and sometimes have really tried to do what they suggest to help myself get healthier. Grow longer and shinier hair in two days. Reverse the aging process. Wish your buttocks away. Eat nothing but pineapples and lose weight, eat nothing but carbs and lose weight, eat nothing but protein and lose weight, eat *nothing*. Let's not forget: lipo yourself to a happier you. Massage therapy, yoga, rolfing, kick boxing—you name it! I have tried giving up meat, and I stopped eating foods high in fat, ate no sugar or salt . . . *boring!* Nothing worked, by the way. However, in the back of my mind—which was way too crowded!—the seeds of a healthier way of life were planted.

Like millions of other people, I have succumbed to the American diet and take great delight in high-fat foods, red meat, and rich, sugary desserts. How was I going to continue eating the foods I *love* without giving up what I really love to eat?

Since I love to cook so much, I have found a way

to eat most of the foods I want so I don't feel deprived. Living in California, where fresh fruits and vegetables are easily available, is a huge advantage. I noticed that when I kept my diet to low-fat, high-fiber foods, I just plain felt better. But I'm weak! I *love* butter and gooey cheeses and potato chips. Ice cream with hot fudge sauce. Great big sandwiches on sourdough or French bread, filled with salami, prosciutto, mortadella, sausage, and peppers! Cream pies, fruit pies, cakes, rich chocolate brownies, M&Ms and peanut butter cups. Italian food, Chinese food, Thai food, French food, any kind of food.

But reality finally hit me. I simply got fed up with not feeling well. I was tired and irritable more often than not. In the morning when I woke, my head hurt with a dull throb in the back of my skull. My whole body ached and felt stiff. The first few steps out of bed were an adventure just to make it to the bathroom. How I longed for the days when I would leap out of bed, walk without creaking, and get dressed without worrying which leg was strong enough to hold me up as I tried to bend to get my pants on.

Also, I had begun to show specific signs of menopause. My periods were sporadic. I was becoming even more irritable, and for the first time I was experiencing anxiety and mild depression. I had my first hot flash at Nieman-Marcus, and initially I thought it was from seeing the bill from my purchases.

I knew in my head what I needed to do. It was making that decision to change. Since my body was going through a change anyway, I had to make adjustments in order to help myself along and stay as healthy as I could for as long as I could. This has not been easy.

IT'S YOUR DECISION

I understood that I needed to make decisions I really didn't want to make. Like giving up certain foods that simply were not good for me.

I had to give up eating butter, chocolate (I have devised a way to eat my chocolate, which I will share with you in the recipe section), red meat, sugar, wine, and caffeine.

I never drank much wine to begin with because every time I did, I would have a negative reaction. I later found out through my nutritionist that I do not assimilate sugar well. I immediately get a dull, throbbing headache in the back of my head and, if this makes sense, in my eyes! Ten to fifteen minutes later I get extremely irritable, then drowsy. If I'm out for dinner with Tony, it's so embarrassing when my head ends up on my plate.

Once Tony and I were with some friends in Acapulco. Every evening around seven o'clock everyone gathered around for margaritas with chips and salsa. They served the drinks in frosty salted glasses, and the contents were slushy, cold, and satisfying! While people around me were slowly sipping theirs, mine was gone in five minutes. Before I knew it, there was another one in front of me. Halfway through that one, I noticed things I hadn't noticed before. Tony had two heads, and everything looked funny to me. And I couldn't get up! Tony gently helped me get back to our room as I was trying to explain to him that watching the sunset would make him go blind. I didn't remember anything after that, except I threw up violently and fell asleep.

I woke up an hour later feeling much better and managed to get myself dressed. (How did I get naked?) We went back for dinner. Everyone was rather quiet, and not making eye contact with me. Finally someone looked at me and said, "Yahoo?"

I said, "Excuse me?"

Evidently they had heard sounds coming from the bedroom, and Tony and I had had a rip-roaring time, as I did things to him that he had never even thought of! I must have thought I was riding a bull at a rodeo. The combination of sugar and alcohol obviously *does not* agree with me. I didn't remember a thing, but Tony sure looked happy!

You should always be aware of how alcohol affects you, mentally and physically. Alcohol is known to irritate the lining of the stomach. The greatest damage is to the liver. Obviously, I don't drink often enough to do any damage to my liver, but my head sure can feel funny. If you do drink even a little, you should be sure you include in your diet extra vitamin B-complex, vitamin C, vitamin E, calcium, zinc, and iron. So says Isadore Rosenfeld, M.D., who wrote a terrific book I highly recommend that you read: *Doctor, What Should I Eat?*

What you put into your body determines how you will feel. The old adage "You are what you eat" is so true! There is just no way around it. Processed foods, refined sugars, and meats upset the natural balance of your metabolism. I truly believe a balanced diet of unprocessed and whole foods along with herbs and vitamin supplements will turn your life around. Eating a vegetarian diet is probably the wisest way to go. But I'm being realistic—I really do enjoy chicken, fish, lamb, an occasional burger, and yes, sometimes a big fat steak!

If you take care of your body in the right way, you can enjoy all of the things you love. I do notice, however, that the more often I eat whole foods, grains, fruits, and vegetables, the more my desire for meat diminishes. When I do eat meat, I can feel the residual effects—stomachaches, bloating, and gas.

HOW TO GET STARTED

Along with dietary changes, I wanted to explore using natural herbs and vitamins to help keep my hormones in balance. I asked my friends, doctors, and a homeopathic pharmacist about herbalists, and I found one who lives close by. It's important to note that at all times I kept all my doctors informed about what I was taking and who suggested that I take it.

Our first meeting lasted two hours as I filled out

a lengthy questionnaire about my medical history. I explained what had brought me to him in the first place—that I was perimenopausal and wanted to help out my body as much as I could the natural way, without having to resort to synthetic hormones. I also explained that I had lost my sex drive, that I knew using just a testosterone cream was not enough, and that I needed to balance my hormones in a nonintrusive way.

What follows is what my herbalist suggested for me and why. *Remember, this program was designed for me based on my own personal medical history. What works for me will probably not be right for you.* A lot of factors need to be included, such as family history of breast and ovarian cancer and heart disease and what kind of medications you are on and why. But you can read the information below to learn more about your options.

ANTIOXIDANTS

Vitamins A, B-complex, C, and E, also called antioxidants, are used to fend off free radicals. Free radicals are molecules generated by cells in the body when it is exposed to toxins, germs, or viruses. Your body produces free radicals in order to protect itself from these invaders. But the cells themselves can become targets of the free radicals and must protect themselves with antioxidants. Antioxidants are enzymes that protect your body by capturing free radicals and escorting them out of your body before they do any damage. When free radicals attack your unprotected cells, they change the molecular structure of the cells. Cells that are damaged become an easy target to weaken your immune system, possibly leading to cancer and other ailments.

The amount of free radicals in your body is directly affected by the food you eat (especially fatty foods), the toxins you breathe, cigarette smoke, and household chemicals and contaminants. In order to protect yourself, you need to take antioxidants.

I take daily doses of the antioxidants beta-carotene, vitamin B-complex, vitamin C, and vitamin E.

Beta-carotene

Beta-carotene is the precursor to vitamin A. It is a carotenoid, a type of pigment found in plants. Your skin stores beta-carotene and your body metabolizes it to produce vitamin A. It increases your resistance to infection. It may help prevent some cancers. Beta-carotene may also help lower cholesterol levels and reduce the risk of heart disease.

I take beta-carotene once a day instead of vitamin A. With beta-carotene, you will safely get all the vitamin A you need, along with antioxidant protection. The only side effect of consuming too much is that your skin might turn yellow. The color will go away in a few weeks if you cut back on your dosage.

WARNING! Please consult your doctor before you take any form of vitamin A. If you are pregnant or suffer from kidney disease it can be toxic.

B-complex

Vitamin B-complex is a combination of eight essential vitamins. Together they can combat stress, depression, and cardiovascular disease. Vitamin B helps your brain, blood, and a lot of your body functions stay in balance. You need it to help your cells grow and reproduce. It helps keep your red blood cells healthy and helps prevent birth defects.

It's important to take all the B vitamins, because each has its own job to do. If you are low on any one, the others cannot do their jobs. The B vitamins all do the larger job of producing energy, making body chemicals such as hormones, and controlling how our cells grow and divide.

Vitamin C

Vitamin C is a powerful antioxidant and immune system booster. Doses of 1,000 mg a day have been suggested for preventing cancer, infections including the common cold, and other ailments.

Vitamin E

Vitamin E accelerates the healing of wounds and protects lung tissue from inhaled pollutants. It may reduce risk for heart disease and prevent premature skin aging. Natural sources of vitamin E are nuts, dark green leafy vegetables, seafood, eggs, and avocados.

MINERALS

Calcium

Calcium is the most abundant mineral in your body, needed to build bones and teeth. It makes some hormones and enzymes, helps your muscles contract, and helps with other functions. Calcium also helps regulate your heartbeat and your blood pressure.

Up to 98 percent of your calcium is in your bones, 1 percent is in your teeth, and 1 percent is in your blood. After about the age of thirty-five, you start to break down bone faster than you can rebuild it. You start to draw on saved-up bone. If you don't get enough calcium, you lose bone mass. Osteoporosis can set in, and your bones start to become thin, brittle, and break very easily.

Magnesium

Along with calcium and phosphorus, magnesium is a main ingredient of bone. A balance of calcium and magnesium is essential for healthy bones and teeth, and reduces the risk of osteoporosis. Calcium and magnesium also help regulate muscle activity. Cal-

cium stimulates contraction; magnesium induces re-
laxation.

Your body especially needs magnesium during
stress or illness. It has really helped me with my pre-
menstrual syndrome and cramps. I also suffered from
leg cramping, which seems to be under control since
I started taking calcium and magnesium.

HERBS AND NUTRITIONAL SUPPLEMENTS

Here's a list of herbs and nutritional supplements I
have incorporated into my life. Some of them I don't
use every day, only when I become aware that my
body is not feeling its best.

Dong Quai

Dong quai is a root used to reduce pain in menstruation and to help establish a regular cycle. It is consid-
ered a very useful herb for all gynecological problems
that are due to deficient, poor-quality, or stagnant
blood. I drink dong quai in a tincture (a few drops in
water) a week to ten days before my period. It seems
to help quiet my nerves, too.

Evening Primrose Oil

This is oil from the seeds of the plant known as evening primrose. The therapeutic component of the oil,
known as gamma-linolenic acid, is an essential fatty

acid. Gamma-linolenic acid supports the body's production of estrogen and progesterone and affects the overall hormone balance. When the supply of gamma-linolenic is deficient, the symptoms of PMS become more pronounced.

I use it for sore breasts. About ten days before my period, my breasts used to become swollen and tender to the touch. I could feel the heaviness and pain constantly, and it was so debilitating. Even wearing clothing was painful.

I didn't notice a difference right after I started taking evening primrose oil. It took four to five months, but I don't have symptoms any longer. I can't tell you what a relief this is. Evening primrose oil comes in capsule form, and I take two in the morning and two at night.

St. John's Wort

St. John's Wort is a flowering herb that can have beneficial effects on various brain disturbances, including depression. About a week before my period I can get so depressed. I cry easily, and my head feels like it's ready to explode. Now I use St. John's Wort in capsule form or in a tincture—twenty to thirty drops in a quarter glass of water—once or twice a day until the onset of my period. It calms me down, and I definitely feel much better.

Mexican Wild Yam

This is an extract taken from the root of the wild yam, a perennial vine. It relaxes the muscles of the entire abdominal region. It is prescribed to relieve menstrual cramps and muscle tension. It also acts as an anti-inflammatory.

I take it in capsule form daily to prevent menstrual discomfort. I also use it in a cream form as a body moisturizer for the progesteronelike properties it supplies. It helps balance my hormones.

Milk Thistle

I take milk thistle for my liver. More about milk thistle in chapter 6.

Ginkgo Biloba

The ginkgo is the world's oldest living species of tree, dating back more than 200 million years. Ginkgo is the herbal medicine most frequently prescribed by alternative-minded doctors worldwide. It has been shown to increase circulation to the brain and the extremities, and to improve circulation in both large vessels (arteries) and small vessels (capillaries).

Research in Europe and elsewhere has shown that the tree leaf extract is also extremely effective in prevention and treatment of early Alzheimer's disease and strokes. By increasing blood flow to the brain, it appears to decrease symptoms such as dizziness and memory loss.

I take it in pill form for my memory.

Psyllium

These ground-up seeds, rich in fiber, help with both diarrhea and constipation, because the herb absorbs excess fluid in the intestinal tract and increases stool volume. It makes a safe, gentle, bulk-forming laxative.

Make sure you drink ten to twelve eight-ounce glasses of water every day while taking psyllium—or even if you're not! Psyllium can just sit there and block everything unless you give it plenty of water.

As a bonus, your skin will look healthier and younger. Water is the secret ingredient. You'll flush everything out, feel so much better, and lose those extra pounds.

CHANGING MY HABITS

I have changed my habits because my old ones were doing me in. It was a conscious decision. I'm eating more soy, fruits, and vegetables. But it was not that easy at first, and I found myself going back to my old way of doing things.

A lot of the problem is just plain inconvenience. Who wants to remember to take all those vitamins and herbs every day? But every time I did forget, I felt the effects right away. Now I carry a plastic compartmentalized box with me. In it I store some of my vitamins with their labels, in case I forget to take them in the morning, or if I'm running late or simply too lazy. I put the box in my bag along with snacks such as fruit, cut-up veggies, rice cakes, pretzels, popcorn, and soy nuts.

Sometimes I simply run out of steam, and my blood sugar level goes so low that I actually have a difficult time trying to put sentences together. I feel light-headed and get a headache. If I don't carry food with me, I inevitably reach for all the wrong foods I shouldn't be eating and end up pigging out. I recognize this in myself, and I've tried to stop the destructive behavior. I am very proud of that!

That doesn't mean I don't slip now and then—I'm only human and I still experience stress—but I don't beat myself up anymore when I do. After all, tomorrow you can start again!

In order for you to understand why I *had* to make these life-altering choices, I have to fill you in on a little background.

3

How Could This Ever Happen to Me?

There I was on the thirty-eighth floor of the ABC building in New York. Little did I know that I had a date with destiny, although you never would have known it from our first meeting. I was there to meet Tony Thomopoulos, the head of the network. Everyone told me what a dashing (yes, they used the word dashing), handsome, and powerful figure he was. Everyone referred to him as the Greek God or the Silver Fox.

I was there to get final approval from the network (that was Tony) for a job at *Good Morning America*.

After I went through a slew of security people, I was escorted upstairs with all these hall passes with my name written all over them. (Just in case I decided to steal the fall lineup, they would know whom to blame.)

I watched the sun set over the buildings in the city as I sat waiting in his office. I waited and waited and waited. Finally, in strolled this magnificent-looking man with a big corporate attitude.

I hated him.

First of all, he didn't even apologize for keeping me waiting forty-five minutes. Then he had this very proper, almost arrogant air about him. Plus, he smirked! I was so annoyed. I quickly announced that I had a car waiting downstairs and dinner reservations that I was late for. He hated me! He treated me like I wasn't even there, very noncommittal. The meeting was strained, although I tried to be my normal, charming self. I could see we were getting nowhere, and he quickly ended the meeting.

Needless to say, I didn't get the job—but I got the man!

How did this one disastrous meeting turn into the best thing that has ever happened to me?

I kept running into Tony after that first meeting, in both New York and Los Angeles. He was always very polite, and still very handsome. After the initial hello-how-are-you-nice-to-see-you-again (yeah, right), he would just ignore me. So why did I find myself so fascinated with this guy? After all, he was married, and so was I.

For the following four years we would casually run

into each other, shake hands, and move on. During that time, Tony and his wife separated and divorced. I was still very much married and going about my life just fine, thank you. Then one evening during dinner, a friend answered the phone and said to me, "Cristina, I think you better take this one." We had a rule in our house (still do): No phone calls during dinner. My friend insisted. I reached for the phone, and the person on the other end announced he was from the *Los Angeles Times* and wanted a quote from me about my then-husband's arrest.

From that moment on my life was changed forever. (I won't go into the details now. Believe me, that's a whole other book.) For the next two years, I tried to keep a semblance of normalcy around my two young children, Zachary and Kathryn. It was a very difficult, tumultuous, upsetting, and sad time. Our marriage couldn't hold up under the strain. As soon as the trial was over, I asked for a divorce. I moved with my two small children to Los Angeles to be near my family.

That is where Tony reentered my life. I was offered a job to host a local talk show called *A.M. Los Angeles* for ABC. So, you guessed it, I needed to get approval from the Big Guy. This time word came back from New York that he had given his approval, and I started my career as a talk show host.

Later, I was invited to go to an ABC function for Aaron Spelling, who was important to the network because he had so many hit shows—*Charlie's Angels,*

Dynasty, and *The Love Boat,* just to name a few. It was there that the sparks started to fly. Tony got up to give a toast to Aaron. But before he said anything, he raised his glass, acknowledged me, and told everyone how much he admired and respected me. (What?!) He went on to say that I had handled the trial with grace and dignity.

I was floored! I looked up at him and he was definitely looking back at me. I swear I had a power surge! I couldn't look at him the rest of the evening because I knew I was in big trouble. He came up to me after the dinner to say to my face everything he had just expressed before.

A few weeks went by and I was invited to go to yet another ABC function. I couldn't get the word yes out fast enough, because I knew *he* would be there.

It was a black tie affair, so I pulled out all the stops. Killer hair, killer makeup, shoes, and dress.

I arrived at the party—and Tony was there with a date! I managed to have a pleasant time in spite of my disappointment. Toward the end of the evening, I found myself sitting all alone at a round table for ten. Everyone was on the dance floor, dancing to this beautiful music under the stars. Finally from this sea of people emerged my fantasy. He stood there looking to-die-for in his tuxedo, his silver hair shimmering in the lights. He looked straight at me. I stared right back at him and said, "Would you care to dance?" He hesitated for a moment and then said, "No." I couldn't believe what I had just heard. No, he said, no! What was with this guy? I could feel myself turning red, starting from my toes. He turned around to walk away, his hands in his pockets. He took a few steps, stopped, then slowly turned around. I swear it was almost surreal, as everything seemed to stop— the music, the evening, my heart. He walked back over to me, extended his hand and said, "I would very much like to dance with you."

By this time I was so confused I didn't know whether to tell him yes or bug off! I found myself automatically getting up from my chair as I took his hand. We went out onto the dance floor. As I raised my arm around his neck, he slid his arm around my waist and brought me in close to him. The minute I touched his body I could smell his cologne. I felt weak in my knees. By the time I got my breath back, the music had stopped. We found ourselves with our arms still wrapped around each other, both of us not wanting to let go, both of us not wanting the moment to end. He escorted me back to the table. Please God, I thought, have him ask for my phone number. Just as I finished my little prayer he asked. I gave it to him gladly.

Tony and I were married six months later. It's been an all-consuming, passionate love affair. We live and breathe for each other. When one of us is away for some reason, he calls me to say that taking a breath is painful when I'm not by his side.

For over fifteen years we have lusted for each

other, making love in every conceivable place we could find. In the beginning I was always shocked by Tony's freedom from any inhibitions. He taught me to have fun and to be free.

I think I may have carried it too far one time. Tony was coming home from business in New York. He had been gone for more than a week, and I wanted to surprise him. So I decided to splurge and hired a stretch limousine to take me to the airport. I wore only high heels and an overcoat. I wasn't concerned about anything until I had to go through the security check. If anything had beeped, I would have died. But I made it through just fine.

Then I was waiting for his plane to arrive. I was a bit uncomfortable, as the terminal was warm. They were very polite in the lounge, and a steward offered to take my coat and bring me a drink. Lucky for me, just then they announced the arrival of Tony's flight. I saw him coming and my heart skipped a beat, just as it always does when I see him. He was smiling and chatting away with someone. As they got closer, I recognized that it was a friend of ours.

After we all greeted one another, Tony announced to me that he had offered our friend a ride home! I couldn't believe it! I'd been sweating in this coat for almost an hour, and now I couldn't even take it off in the car. Tony then said, "Gee, honey, aren't you hot? Here, let me take your coat." I insisted that I was fine, but just then he pulled open the front. When he realized I had nothing on underneath, he quickly closed me up and whispered, "Are you crazy?!" He wasn't angry—he thought it was great!

Now he couldn't figure out how to get rid of our friend. He was so disappointed that he wasn't able to do anything on the way home. Especially since every time our friend wasn't looking, I would flash Tony, which made him nuts! Well, all I can say is we ended up dropping our friend off at the corner of his street, not even at his house.

Tony and I have always enjoyed one another with great gusto and humor. He taught me to like and accept myself, whether I was thin, pregnant, or simply overweight. He always made me feel as if I was the sexiest woman in the world. I knew he wanted me anyway and always, and that made me feel loved. I always responded happily whenever he would want to make love.

Then I started to notice a change.

4

Okay, So I Don't Have a Headache

Tony and I went from having sex three to four times a week to once every week, then once every ten days to two weeks. I was starting to make up excuses not to make love. Every time Tony reached for me, I would give him some dumb reason not to do it. He finally said that maybe I should get an X ray of my head if I kept having all these headaches. *Okay, so I don't have a headache. I just don't want to have sex.*

I noticed a difference in my libido about two years ago and never gave it much thought. I just figured the stress of running a home, taking care of a husband and children, and managing a career had finally got to me. Especially since I had started *Home and*

Family, a two-hour show we ran live every day, Monday through Friday, from 1996 to 1998.

In the beginning it was a challenge for everyone, as we were starting up a brand-new production. I would get up at five o'clock three days a week to do my exercises. (If I don't do them then, it's totally impossible for me to do them at all.) When I was done, I would run upstairs to shower and get dressed. Then I would help get the kids up for school as I listened to all the reasons they couldn't go to school that morning. I would gently feel their foreheads and say, "If you don't have a fever of at least one-oh-five, you have to go to school!" With that out of the way, I headed downstairs to make sure their lunch was packed and breakfast was on the table.

I must say that I am extremely blessed. I have had the same wonderful, heaven-sent women helping me with my children and house ever since Alexandra was born twelve years ago. I don't know how I would be able to work and have peace of mind without Birdie and Irene. They bring us nothing but joy. If I didn't have them in my life, there's absolutely no way I could do everything. Tony, the children, and I are forever grateful. I have so much respect for all women who manage to do it all without any help!

After I would go over the day's schedule with Birdie and Tony—who has drama, who has soccer, what time should they get picked up, any doctor or dentist appointments, and so on and so on—I would head for the studio. I was there by 7:30. There was always a ton of things waiting for me to go through when I arrived. I would sit down with my assistant to take care of everything and schedule my day. Then I wrote thank-you notes to all the guests from the week before. After I caught up on all the gossip, I would start to write letters in the makeup chair. When I was all pulled together, I would rehearse that day's show. Then back to my trailer, where I would usually go through three or four outfits before I settled on one.

We would start live at ten o'clock each day, finishing at noon. During that time I had to be on top of my game. There wasn't any down time. After the show was over I always felt happy and energized, since I love what I do and the people I work with.

After the show, I would go over the next day's show one more time with the staff. Then I returned phone calls and went off to do my errands, like grocery shopping or taking care of whatever extra business I had before the kids came home from school around 3:30. Then came snack time, followed by plenty of homework. Between Alex and Arianna I have now repeated elementary school.

After homework I started to prepare dinner. (I'm usually spent by eight o'clock, but that hour is very important to me because this is when I can really be with the girls without homework and chores hanging over their heads.) When nine o'clock came, it was time for bed, and I get to hear all the reasons they don't want to go to sleep. When they were finally settled down, I had to wait a good forty-five minutes, because inevitably they would get up six times to tell me something they'd forgotten. Or they were thirsty or hungry, or a report was due the next day. When they were finally asleep, Tony wanted to have his time with me. By that time I was like a sponge that has been oversaturated. I just couldn't take in any more. I sat there and tried to be interested, but I was like a zombie.

One night after more than a week without sex, Tony simply looked at me and said, "I see. No sex now for the rest of my life, right?" I felt like a failure. Those words really hurt me, but I didn't care. I was just so tired, the thought of having sex was painful to me.

I figured all right, I'll try and get some extra sleep. That didn't work. We took a little weekend getaway. That didn't work, either. I simply resigned myself to the fact that my sexual desire had gone, and I just had to find a way to accommodate Tony. Yes, I said accommodate. I would actually count the evenings that would go by. After so many days I figured I'd better, or there'd be trouble in paradise.

5

PMS, Stress, and Menopause

I suffered for many years from PMS. Ever since the birth of my last child eight years ago, it really escalated. About ten days before the onset of my period, I would start to become more irritable. Then came the crying jags and depression. I would overreact to the littlest things. My hearing would become so acute that the sound of a utensil falling on the floor would have the same effect as putting my head inside the Liberty Bell! My breasts were so tender and swollen that taking a shower, not to mention wearing clothes, was painful. I was irritable with the kids and wanted to shoot my husband. Especially if he wanted to have sex. *Forget about it!*

Something would go terribly wrong two to three days before I started my period. I would tear the house apart looking for some chocolate. Stock in

M&M/Mars and Reese's would go up as I would consume massive quantities of M&Ms and peanut butter
cups. And I don't even usually like sweets! But if
I couldn't find some in the special treat drawer, I
would raid the children's lunch boxes, hoping I
would find a morsel of some kind. It finally got so
bad that I would keep a stash hidden away just for
these insane times.

One time I went so far as to actually hide seven
packets of peanut butter cups in my bra, so my husband wouldn't catch me with all that chocolate. *I had
to have it!* I devised a way to get all this candy by him.
I went quietly downstairs to the kitchen, where I hid
my treasures, and carefully unwrapped each package.
(I even got rid of the candy wrappers by squishing
them together, wrapping toilet paper around the
wad, and tossing it in the garbage.)

Then I quickly stuffed the candy in my bra, closed
up my robe, and very nonchalantly headed up the
stairs as if butter, or should I say chocolate, wouldn't
melt in my mouth. I casually walked by my husband
and asked him how his day was, knowing full well I
was standing there with 4,000 calories in my bra. All
the while I'm thinking to myself, "Ha, I really fooled
this guy!" If I had put the candy in my bra still
wrapped, the rattling of the paper would have given
me away! God forbid if he tried to hug me!

Then I ate the candy in a bizarre ritual. I went into
my bathroom, locked the door, of course, and filled
up my tub with a hot bubble bath. I took the soft
peanut butter cups out and lined them up ever so

strategically along the side of the tub, got into my cozy bath, and ate each one just as I eat Ritz crackers, starting at one end of the rim and going in a circular motion until they all disappeared, relishing every moment. After I consumed all fourteen of them I went into a diabetic shock! (Not really.)

Although I didn't binge like that all the time, I still ate a lot of chocolate. I couldn't get over how the chocolate would be so calming, at least for a while. Then, when I went to bed, I would have such a sugar high I'm surprised I could stay still, let alone fall asleep.

The next morning would always be hell. I'd wake up with such a hangover! My head would hurt and my body would ache. I would be in such a horrible, nasty mood, I didn't know who to yell at first. I would swear that this was the absolute last time I would binge like this . . . and I would keep my word, until the next month.

Why did I do this to myself, my family, my co-workers, the world? What force was behind me making me make these wrong choices? Why couldn't I control it? What was happening to my body at this particular time of the month to make me do such irrational and destructive things to myself?

PREMONSTRAL SYNDROME

The research I did on PMS—which Tony has so lovingly dubbed pre*monstral* syndrome—has helped me in finding the answers to these questions.

At least 60 percent of all women suffer from PMS at some time in their lives. It is most likely to occur in their thirties, though it can occur as early as adolescence and as late as the perimenopausal years.

If you know your body well, or if you keep a chart for at least three months, you will see a definite pattern to PMS (Tony, in the interest of keeping our relationship intact, figured out when I had turned the corner to the other side. He knew he had a four- to five-day window every month when he could actually talk to me without my breaking down crying if he said good morning the wrong way.)

There are more than a hundred known symptoms of PMS. Here are the ones I've dealt with:

- abdominal bloating
- abdominal cramps
- aggression
- back pain
- alcohol intolerance
- anxiety
- breasts swelling and becoming tender to the touch
- depression
- emotional overreaction
- food binges
- hives
- irritability
- rage
- sex drive changes

- cravings for sweets
- despondency (over what, I don't know)

My symptoms would start, then escalate over the seven to ten days before my period, then stop abruptly when I started to bleed.

I read almost every book I could get my hands on to understand what I could do to help myself get over this major problem in my life. I was forty-six, and with menopause staring me in the face I was even more concerned. There is a ton of information out there, so I tried to identify the most important factors and simplify them. I began with the factors that affect hormone levels.

As I researched further I found out that many things affect hormone levels. The food you eat, the air you breathe, driving, the kids, your job, husband, boyfriend, boss, parents, school—just everyday, ordinary living. It's called *stress!*

STRESS

We all experience stress. There's good stress and bad stress.

According to Dr. Susan Love, one of the foremost experts on breast cancer, "One of the worst threats to health is chronic stress. It increases blood pressure, respiratory rate, heart rate, and oxygen consumption." Chronic stress can lead to heart disease, high blood pressure, and cancer.

Stressful situations are all around us, and we cannot always avoid them. But no matter what kind of stress you have, it affects your body and how it functions. You need to learn how to be aware of your stress levels, and most important, how to manage them.

Remember the last time you took a vacation? I am not a good traveler. In fact, I hate it! I'm afraid to fly, so that causes major anxiety. I don't like crowds, and I have a major problem with public restrooms, although I do have the strongest thighs in the world from doing squats.

At the airport, everyone is always frowning. Traveling is stressful enough, then you add to it by eating airline food that causes more stress as your body tries to digest all the sugar, salt, and processed ingredients.

I'm always amused and somewhat confused when they announce that your flight is boarding and everyone rushes to be the first one on the plane—as if it's going to take off without them! They rush and then wait forever, inching along in that tubular jetway, just to sit in the plane as they load two hundred more passengers. God forbid if someone cuts in the line. People are so tense that they actually become indignant, staring at you with looks to kill and saying, with voice full of sarcasm, "Uh, excuse me, but I was here first." *What difference does it make?*

Then there's airplane food. What can I say? *Nothing* available to eat even remotely looks like food. You end up looking over at the other passengers to see what they got. Now you're aggravated because their food actually looks better than yours!

So there you are, stuffed into these seats, and there's always a crying baby somewhere. People are coughing or sneezing and don't even bother to cover their mouths. And the restroom always has drops of urine on the toilet seat and the floor! I have to roll up my pants to my thighs so the hems don't touch the floor. I can't take it. Major stress!

Then there is getting off the plane after it lands. You're in an even worse mood than when you started, plus you have dried-out nasal passages. Everyone quickly grabs all of their belongings in a desperate attempt to be at the door when it opens. You stand with everyone on top of you for at least five minutes, waiting to burst out the door the second it opens. Sometimes it takes a lot longer, especially if you get someone who does not know how to operate the jetway. You watch helplessly as they try to maneuver this thing back and forth, left to right, up and down. I actually get seasick as I watch it weaving in and out in an attempt to connect with the door. When it finally does, do they let you out? Of course not! They have to have this little conversation and exchange paperwork before they step aside. When they do, everyone rushes out the door to be the first one at the luggage area—only to wait forty-five minutes for their bags.

I was detained once for over an hour because I lost one claim ticket. Normally I would understand this, since a lot of bags look alike and all that. But it was Christmas, and after numerous delays because of bad weather, I finally arrived in Los Angeles eleven hours after we were supposed to take off from New York— with two of those screaming kids I talked about before (mine, I confess) and ten pieces of cheap matching luggage. I had decided that year I was going to do all my Christmas shopping in New York and bring all the gifts along with me. (I was trying to save shipping costs—what an idiot!) The bags were all black nylon with a big fat red stripe. I finally got them all together after waiting until the very end for the last two. I started out the door but got stopped because I had lost one of the claim checks along the way (probably when I was rolling up my pants in the john). I was told I had to produce the claim check or else they would not let me leave with one of the ten pieces of luggage. "Excuse me," I said in my most controlled voice, "but do you see the other *nine* pieces of luggage that match? Does that give you any clue?" But they didn't budge, even though there were literally hundreds of people behind me trying to get through! I had two kids, ten bags, and one extremely angry man (my husband) alongside me as I tried to explain to the head claims manager that if there were nine pieces of matching black luggage with a *big fat red stripe* down the middle, the tenth piece was most likely mine as well! Finally I was released. Aaarrrgg-ghhh! No wonder your body gives you signals. It's on total overload.

ROAD RAGE

Of course, you don't need to travel by plane to add stress to your daily routine. All you have to do is get into your car. Who knows what adventures await you there?

I have a couple of questions. Why is it when you put on your blinkers to change lanes, people automatically speed up? Aren't they supposed to let you in? Why, if a car stops in front of you to turn left and you want to get into the right lane to pass, do the people in back of you honk and scream as they whiz by you, call you a jerk, and give you the finger? Weren't you in front of them in the first place?

Road rage! Thank God I only suffer from it once a month! When I'm in the PMS mode, no one is safe. That's why I firmly believe that it's important to control these violent mood swings. I realize my behavior is totally inappropriate, and I cannot let hormonal rage control me.

The turning point for me came when I was at a stoplight. There were two cars in front of me, a car to my left, and a car to my right. Someone behind me in this beat-up white truck honked his horn. I look in my rearview mirror and he signaled me to move up. Move up? Where? He honked again. I ignored him. Next thing I know, he tapped my bumper and started pushing my car forward.

You do not do this when a woman is not one with her body. I slammed hard on my brakes, put the car in park, and opened my door. I went over to him and started in on him like he had just run over my dog. I used such foul language that I had to ground myself when I got home. He started to go at me, but I guess I scared him so much, he got this strange look on his face and rolled up the window.

The light changed and he took off. Did I stop there and just let it go? Why should I? I was Raging Hormone Woman, put on the streets to stop rude people on the road. I quickly got back into my car and went after him. I finally caught up and cut him off. He came to a stop. I got out of the car, this time with my magic weapon—the cellular phone! I quickly announced that he had messed with the wrong woman. I told him that I had phoned the police and reported his license plates, that he had better get off the road immediately because they were coming to get him. He took off like a shot again. This time I let him go.

That night, when Tony got home, I told what had happened. I really didn't feel good about my behavior. He was angry with me for taking such a chance and getting out of the car in the first place. He said, "Are you crazy? You could have been shot or run over. I certainly would have run you over. Cristina, you need to get hold of yourself. You need to control your irrational behavior."

He is so right, but sometimes I can't control the way I feel and react to things. I have different reactions to everything. You never know which incident will set me off. The time of the month determines my reactions. In the middle of my cycle I can handle anything with reason and relative calm. But other times I can't take the smallest inconvenience.

PHONING IT IN

Here's another example. I went to a department store to buy bedding. First, you can't find anyone to help you. Somehow they're always in the towel department on the other side of the store! You start to rummage through the endless packages of mismatched sheets and always end up with one package you can't find, like the fitted bottom sheet.

When you finally do find someone and ask her to help, she inevitably goes through the same batch of sheets you have already been through twice. Reluctantly she heads to the back storage room to see if she can locate it for you. You pace back and forth waiting for her, and fifteen minutes later she finally emerges. In the meantime, because you're bored, you find another set of sheets you really, really like, on sale. You buy them, but of course you can't find the standard-size pillowcases. So your salesperson disappears into the back room again. She comes out fifteen minutes later, but this time you just want out! As she starts to add up your bill, the phone rings, and she answers it. She starts to help the person on the phone. After she looks up what the person on the phone wants, she continues with your order, only to be interrupted once again by the phone.

But one time I reached over and actually took the phone from the clerk and announced to the caller that the clerk would call back at a later time. I explained as calmly as I could that I actually got in my car, drove all the way to the store, and picked out the merchandise myself. If I thought that I could have just *phoned it in,* I would have saved myself all that time!

Now, I am not proud of my reactions. I am acutely aware that they were wrong. There is no excuse for rude behavior. But I was in a downward spiral and I needed help. As I write this book, I relive everything, and I'm newly horrified at what kind of person I must have been to live with. I don't want to be this way.

KIDS

The worst prospect to me is I still have another set of teenagers to live through! I am convinced if children came into the world as teenagers, no one would have kids! That's where worry, anger, guilt, anxiety, and fear get hold of you, and you live in a constant state of flux.

When they put that little miracle in your arms for the very first time, your first words are not "Gee, I wonder how I can screw up your life?" No, they are these adorable darlings that you would give your life for, and you want to make their lives beautiful. Indeed, the bond between parent and child is so strong that the thought of them not being in your life in mutually loving circumstances is inconceivable!

Then they become teenagers. I can only assume that this is God's way of breaking that strong bond so you can let go.

One evening my son Zachary, who was then sixteen with sandy-colored hair, came home for dinner with a platinum blond buzz cut, the top of his hair shaped into spikes. He walked in with attitude. He strutted around the kitchen waiting for a reaction. I simply looked at him. He walked over to me, started bobbing his head up and down, and said, "What?"

I said, "What?! I'll tell you what. You go back to wherever you just came from and find your hair! You may not return to this house until you do."

Scary words for a mother to say, especially when the kid has car keys. It was a long night. (He showed up several hours later with his original hair color.)

Another time, when my daughter Kathryn was sixteen (a time for major stress on any parent), she was supposed to be home at ten o'clock. Ten o'clock arrived, no Kathryn. All right, I thought, it's okay if she's not right on the nose. Ten-thirty came and went. I started to get concerned. Eleven o'clock, and now I was angry. Eleven forty-five: I was so angry and upset that I was going to ground her for the rest of her life! Midnight: I found myself rocking back and forth on the stairs, making bargains with God. Twelve-twenty: I heard the car coming into the driveway.

My anger was so overwhelming that I knew I was going to lose it right there in the driveway, and the whole neighborhood was going to hear. I opened the door and when I finally saw her emerge from the car, my reaction was not anger but relief. I was so relieved to see that she was okay that I broke down and started sobbing. Kathryn was taken aback. She was visibly shaken and felt so bad that she had worried me. She apologized profusely and swore she would never ever be late again. She never was.

I don't know if being perimenopausal and having teenagers go together. That's why I'm doing everything in my power to make these changes. Not only for my children, but for my most patient and loving husband. And, oh yes, everyone else around me!

FOOD AND EXERCISE

A variety of nutritional factors can contribute to PMS. Various studies have shown that women with PMS tend to have the following nutritional and physiological characteristics:

- high consumption of dairy products
- excessive consumption of caffeine, in the form of soft drinks, coffee, or chocolate
- a relatively high blood level of estrogen, resulting from overproduction from dietary fat or in body fat, or decreased breakdown of estrogen in the liver

High estrogen levels are associated with deficiencies of the vitamin B-complex, especially B6 and B12.

The liver requires these vitamins in order to break down and deactivate estrogen. Also, certain levels of vitamin C, vitamin E, and selenium are required to metabolize estrogen properly.

Chocolate cravings have been linked to low magnesium levels. (I must have no magnesium at all.) The liver needs magnesium along with B vitamins to metabolize estrogen.

I began to pay particular attention to how different foods affected my general well-being. When I ate a balanced diet of fresh fruits and vegetables, protein, and carbohydrates, I was at the top of my game. My body felt in complete harmony as I ate a balanced diet, drank plenty of water, and got regular exercise.

Let me give you an example of how food and exercise can make a difference. I have been extremely fortunate to have had the opportunity to go to the The Golden Door, a slice of heaven nestled in the hills of Escondido, California. In my opinion, it is the finest health spa anywhere. I always come away with more knowledge of how organic food and exercise benefit your well-being.

You arrive on a Sunday to spend the week. On the first evening, everyone congregates in the dining room for dinner. It's always interesting to see how wound-up everyone is.

I remember one year, after the evening meal, the staff gave us a blank sheet of paper and some crayons. They asked us to draw a picture of anything we wanted, using any colors we wanted. After we did, they collected them and simply put them away. After the week was over they brought us out another blank piece of paper and asked us again to draw anything we wanted, using any colors we wanted. This time they brought out the papers we drew at the beginning of the week and asked us to compare them. Well, all I can say is, who in the world drew that first picture? The difference was night and day! We compared our drawings, and we were all astonished at how completely different they were. My first drawing was going in several different directions at once. The colors were gray and the picture was rather bleak. Was this how I was really feeling inside? The second one was of a house, trees, flowers, birds, grass, and a lot of blue sky.

This exercise showed us how we have a brighter outlook and function at a much higher level when we are in harmony with our minds and body. When everyone first arrived at the spa, they had so much excess baggage—and I don't mean suitcases.

I usually go to The Golden Door the second week in January. After the major stress of the holidays, I feel this will help me get a grip.

The first day is not so difficult. You have all the intentions in the world that you are going to get the most of this experience, and you go all out. You start out at six in the morning with a three-mile mountain walk, followed by a delicious breakfast of fresh fruit, juice, and an egg white omelet or cereal. At nine o'clock there is a fifty-minute aerobics class, then a fifty-minute water exercise class. The rest of the day is filled with every kind of class or exercise you can think of: stretching, weights, Stairmaster, treadmill, and so on. Sandwiched between these intense classes are herbal wraps, facials, massages, yoga, and body scrubs.

Of course, when I get out of bed Tuesday morning, I'm totally crippled from overdoing everything! So much for pacing myself. I'm sore and hungry, even though the meals are exquisitely prepared and they feed you extremely well. The executive chef, Michel Stroot, is a genius when it comes to preparing the most delicious, well-planned, beautifully prepared dishes. The philosophy behind The Golden Door, instilled by its founder, Deborah Szekely, over thirty years ago, still holds true today: Taking care of your mind and body through proper nutrition and exercise is the key to optimum health.

By Wednesday, I want to die!

Then something magical happens on Thursday. All that hard work—the hiking, the water exercise, free weights, aerobics, eating healthily, and detoxing—start to pay off. You turn the corner and you are one with your body. Everything starts to change. Your body is starting to get toned, and you like the way it's looking. Your head is clear, because there's nothing to fill it up except fresh air, blood to the brain, and good, clean, healthy food. On my morning hikes I start to really notice and appreciate my surroundings. I feel extremely sensual and can't wait to get home to Tony!

Of course you can't live your everyday life in a spa. But there are little things that you can do at home to help you incorporate a little of that magic.

You are just going to have to take some time out of every day, whether it is ten or fifteen minutes, or one hour. It is vital that you spend some time on yourself to rejuvenate. There are no excuses, not anymore. This is just too important for your health! See chapter 7 for some ideas.

6

Hormones and Life's Energy Flow

Since stress directly affects the balance of our hormones, how do we keep it in check? There's no definitive answer. But I've found several ways to control my mood swings, anxiety, and, yes, sexual desire.

What is a hormone? *Webster's* definition: a chemical substance formed in some organ of the body, such as the adrenal gland or the pituitary gland, and carried to another organ or tissue where it has a specific effect.

The most important factors in helping your body stay balanced are the proper functioning of the liver, the kidneys and adrenals, the pituitary gland, and the thyroid, which will in turn keep your levels of estrogen and progesterone balanced. I found that Paul Pitchford's book *Healing with Whole Foods* was very useful in helping me understand how the various parts of the body work together in harmony. I recommend it for further reading.

Let's talk about hormones first, because they receive most of the attention in discussions of changes at mid-life.

ESTROGEN

Estrogen is a sex hormone that is produced naturally in a woman's body. It includes estradiol (the most potent estrogen in humans), estriol (a relatively weak human estrogen), and estrone (an estrogen produced during pregnancy). It can be found in human placenta, palm kernel oil, and other sources, and can also be prepared synthetically.

As young women, we naturally produce these hormones. I won't give you a lecture on how your body works. If you are perimenopausal then you have been through a thousand periods and know how hormones, or lack thereof, affect your body.

When we were girls, our mothers would sit us down and explain to us what was happening to our bodies. Even though, thank God, there are plenty of books out there to guide us in talking to our own daughters, there's really no one out there talking to us Baby Boomers. So I feel it is important to say that we can empower ourselves to make the right choices, that there are alternatives, and that we needn't be apprehensive about going through the change. It's a natural process, another rite of passage.

Women need estrogen. While research suggests that estrogen is needed to protect hearts and bones, other studies have shown the possibilities of increased risk of breast cancer from too much estrogen. A woman's lifetime risk of breast cancer is one in eight, and if she has a mother or sister who has had breast cancer, it is even higher. While hormone replacement therapy appears to help lessen the risk of heart disease and osteoporosis, other problems can arise, such as increased risk of liver and gallbladder disease, high blood pressure, fibroid tumors, diabetes, and blood clots.

I decided long ago that when the time came I did not want to go on synthetic hormones. I watched my grandmother and my mother struggle for years as they tried to regulate their hormone replacement therapy (HRT), and they were miserable, suffering from headaches, insomnia, irritability, bloating, skin changes, and mood swings. I swore I was not going to be in that same predicament.

When I heard that Premarin, a popular form of estrogen, was manufactured from the urine of pregnant mares, I went whoa—pardon the pun—I don't think I want that inside me! I wanted to take the alternative, natural approach.

Still, alternative therapy requires a big commitment on your part. Hormone replacement therapy is attractive to some woman because it's a whole lot faster and easier to take a pill, and it takes less time to get results. Though I'm concerned with the side effects of HRT, such as a possible increased risk of breast cancer, I'm also afraid of doing nothing, because of the increased risk of heart disease and osteoporosis. But doctors who understand and promote alternative methods will take your diet and lifestyle changes seriously.

One of the facts that keeps coming up in my research is the need for proper diet and exercise to help regulate hormonal levels and keep in good general health.

WHAT KINDS OF FOODS

Natural plant estrogens can be found in certain foods, especially soy and soy products. These phytoestrogens can mimic the effect of your body's own estrogen and lessen menopausal systems, although they don't give us the effect of the hormonal levels we had before menopause.

Please don't be turned off by the fact you are going to have to eat tofu. It is the richest source of protein and natural estrogens. I promise you will love the recipes that I make with tofu. I tried tofu on my kids for a few weeks without telling them, while I was experimenting with recipes for this book. They asked for seconds each time, not knowing a thing. I finally told them what I had been doing because I wanted their honest reactions. They were surprised and shocked, but both of them really liked what I served—delicious, savory, nonfat creamy soups; frosty, thick, nonfat fruit shakes; and lasagna!

Soy and flaxseed contain larger amounts of plant estrogens than any other foods. New research has shown that by eating soy and flaxseed you may enjoy the benefits of estrogen while decreasing the risk of breast cancer.

Consumption of soy products seems to be the reason why women in Japan have fewer menopausal symptoms—only 10 to 15 percent in Japan versus 80 to 85 percent in the United States—as well as a lower rate of breast cancer than women in the United States.

My hero Dr. Andrew Weil suggests eating soy products and flaxseed for their anticancer benefits. Flaxseed can be sprinkled on soups and salads, mixed into drinks and other food, and taken in capsule form.

PROGESTERONE

Progesterone is a hormone manufactured by your ovaries. During your perimenopausal years, the cyclic increase and decrease in progesterone triggers the endometrial shedding known as a menstrual period. When your body produces abnormal levels of progesterone, your menstrual cycles will become irregular.

For those on hormone replacement therapy, studies have shown that taking progestins along with estrogen for at least ten days each month reduces the incidence of uterine cancer. The use of progesterone in hormone replacement therapy can restore the natural estrogen/progesterone balance in a woman's body. Because progesterone has a beneficial effect on the uterus, adding progesterone to HRT reduces the risk of endometrial and uterine cancer caused by excessive estrogen.

As I mentioned in chapter 2, I use natural progesterone cream made from the Mexican wild yam root. I rub a quarter teaspoon on my inner thighs and sometimes my stomach. It has been shown that bone density increases significantly in patients using natural progesterone along with diet and exercise.

OSTEOPOROSIS

One of the things that concerns me the most is osteoporosis, loss of bone mass. *Osteo* means "bone" and *porosis* means "porous," and the term refers to bones that are thin, fragile, and easily broken because they do not contain enough calcium. Until age thirty-five, you build bone mass, but after age thirty-five your bone density starts to decrease. Osteoporotic bones can fracture spontaneously, for no apparent reason. As much as 50 percent of bone mass can be lost by the time a woman reaches menopause.

Preventing Bone Loss

Women need to realize that calcium tablets and estrogen are only a part of building healthy bones. Magnesium, boron, and vitamins D and C are necessary. So are a good diet, stress reduction, and weight-bearing exercise, such as running, weight-training, and step aerobics. I can't say that too many times. Weight-bearing exercise not only prevents bone loss, it has been shown to stimulate the formation of new bone in women who have low bone density.

Smoking and drinking excessive amounts of alcohol contribute to bone loss. Other factors are lack of exercise and a diet high in refined carbohydrates. If you have never given birth, you are also at risk.

The best way to determine your current bone density is through a screening called dual-energy X ray absorptiometry (DEXA). Many doctors (including my own) suggest that you should have this test if you are approaching or in menopause, especially if you have risk factors for osteoporosis. Experts believe the risks of developing breast or uterine cancer, heart disease, and osteoporosis can be traced through your family history. Risks can also be affected by your age, diet, lifestyle, and the kind of replacement hormones you take.

WHAT TO EXPECT

Here is a list of things you can expect when you go through the change:

- hot flashes
- fluid retention
- skin changes

- thinning of hair
- lack of energy
- vaginal dryness and atrophy
- bladder problems
- spotting
- thinning of uterine wall and cervix
- insomnia
- nervousness
- leg cramps
- nosebleeds
- frequent bruising

We've already discussed bone loss. And, of course, lack of sexual desire. Who could blame you? With all this going on, who wants their partner to get close! Whether or not you are on HRT or alternatives, you must be aware of how your cardiovascular system can be affected. You can become more susceptible to heart disease.

WHAT'S A WOMAN TO DO?

You should definitely talk with your doctor about your menopausal symptoms and seek solutions together. Here are some suggestions that helped me through the symptoms I found most troublesome.

Hot Flashes

Hot flashes are characterized by a sudden rush of hot energy, particularly around the head and neck. You may experience sweating, heart palpitations, and a damp feeling on the skin. About 50 to 85 percent of women are affected at some time. About 10 percent of women never experience them at all, while some women experience hourly waves of heat and sweats that totally disrupt their activities, including sleep. This can cause loss of energy and depression.

Hot flashes are related to the erratic production of estrogen (or lack of production) by the ovaries. The actual cause of hot flashes is not known, although it has been theorized that the central thermostat in our brain reacts to a lack of estrogen and causes changes in our body temperature. Hot flashes can last about three to five minutes. You can tell they are coming on for about two to four minutes, then you start to feel the surge, followed by a sudden, hot feeling that spreads upward from your chest and through your body.

Hot flashes usually occur at night, waking you up. One evening I had a glass of red wine with dinner. That night after falling asleep I woke up soaking wet and hot. I was experiencing my first hot flash. I did not like it at all! I mentioned the alcohol because when I spoke to Dr. Reichman, she asked if I had had any wine with dinner. She said alcoholic beverages, hot liquids, spicy food—which I love—and stressful situations cause hot flashes. I might as well move off the planet!

Recently Tony and I renewed our wedding vows. We were remarried in the Greek Church, and it was a very festive occasion. All the people who are dear in our lives were there to share our special day. I felt like a new bride. I truly got all caught up in the moment, from designing the invitations to the dessert reception.

What made it extra-special was that our children participated. Alexandra and Arianna walked down the aisle with our two-year-old granddaughter, Claire, the daughter of Tony's daughter Anne. My father walked me down the aisle, but not before turning to me and saying, "You know, I'm getting tired of doing this with you." (He walked me down the aisle before I married Tony. Twice!) As the door swung open and I heard the beautiful music, I could see in the distance all the people in my life that meant a lot to me, including my husband, who was fighting back tears just like the first time. I waited for the girls to make their way down the aisle, Claire hopping and strutting as if she knew what she was doing.

As I stood there in my knee-length white wool suit with my heart full, I suddenly felt this warm, unmistakable flush envelop my whole body. Oh, God, no! I was suddenly wet all over, and I felt panic. How can I walk down the aisle with beads of sweat all over me? Never in my worst nightmare did I think that I would have hot flashes while I recited my wedding vows. I wanted to wait a few moments so that I could calm down, but the man who coordinates the music to your walking was giving me a gentle shove. By golly, you've got to move on cue! (They're so serious.) I started walking down the aisle.

As I knew this would be the very last time I would be doing this—relax, Dad—I wanted to savor every step, every moment. I wanted to remember every face that leaned forward to smile at me as I passed. I gently wiped the beads of sweat from my brow, my temples, my cheeks, my upper lip, and my neck, knowing that I couldn't get to my back and underneath my breasts and hoping that no one would notice. What I really needed was a bath towel. I managed to reach Tony, and he took my hand and walked me to the altar. We stood there with our children renewing our vows, with me shedding water.

I experienced hot flashes three more times that evening: once more at the church and twice at the reception. I couldn't really enjoy myself, especially with the great Greek dancing, because I was just so darned hot. I kept going outside to stand in the cool ocean breeze. I remember at one point looking up at the sky with my arms outstretched and saying, "There has to be a solution!"

Hormone replacement therapy usually stops the hot flashes. However, I prefer taking natural supplements and eating a diet rich in soy, and it seems to work quite well for me. I have also found that it helps to eat cooling foods such as apples, celery, carrots, alfalfa sprouts, and cucumbers. In his wonderful book *Healing with Whole Foods,* Paul Pitchford recommends eating wheat germ and oils, mung beans, string beans, black beans, and barley for menopausal symptoms in general.

Some supplements used for treating the discomfort of hot flashes include vitamins E, B-complex, C, and A, and calcium with magnesium. (I usually take the calcium with magnesium at night before I go to sleep.) I take vitamin E twice a day, 400 I.U. with meals, for the benefit of my cardiovascular system.

One-fifth of an average block of tofu eaten every day has also been shown to decrease the intensity of hot flashes. Soy and soy products contain phytoestrogens (plant estrogens) and isoflavones, which have been shown to decrease menopausal symptoms and modulate estrogen levels. Some herbs that you can use to help with hot flashes are ginseng, damiana, wild yam, dong quai, passionflower, and sarsaparilla.

Black cohosh is a root containing substances that act like estrogen. A substantial number of controlled clinical trials have shown that black cohosh improves vaginal lubrication and reduces depression, headaches, and hot flashes. Black cohosh also acts as a sedative. You may have to use black cohosh for at least four to six weeks before you experience any results. Black cohosh can cause serious side effects. See your doctor before taking it.

I must say this again: Don't just read this information and say, okay let me try these and see what happens. Find a doctor who knows about alternative medicine. There are some herbs and vitamins I take that perhaps, for whatever reason, you shouldn't. For instance, ginseng helped me with my hot flashes and sex drive, but if you have hay fever, fibrocystic breasts, asthma, emphysema, high blood pressure, blood clotting problems, heart disorder, or diabetes, you must be under the care of a herbalist or licensed health-care professional if you want to take it. If you are going to turn to alternative ways to help you through menopause, you must seek out advice of experts.

Vaginal Dryness

What a turnoff. What happened? I can't believe how uncomfortable it became to have sex. I swear I felt like a shriveled-up prune as my husband, being ever so supportive, told me how he loved and adored me as he tried to maneuver his way. It made me feel *awful!*

Vaginal dryness is caused by the decreased hormone production that occurs during menopause. The vaginal lining contains glands that secrete fluid when stimulated by hormones produced by the ovaries. The supplements we have discussed for hot flashes help with vaginal dryness as well. Herbs such as dandelion leaves and oat straw, taken orally, have also been used to restore vaginal lubrication. Aloe vera gel can be used as a lubricant.

The 2 percent testosterone vaginal cream I use every third or fourth day helps me tremendously with that problem. Remember, I was tested and found to have a very low testosterone level, which also accounted for my low sex drive.

Loss of Sex Drive

Well, I guess I'm an expert on this subject.

At least 50 percent of menopausal women report no decline in sexual interest, and fewer than 20 percent report any significant decline—although judging from the overwhelming response I got from the my appearances on *Dateline* and *Oprah,* I thought it was the whole country!

Loss of sexual desire during menopause does not usually result from loss of hormone production. Masters and Johnson have shown that the sex drive is not related to estrogen levels and therefore should not automatically decline with menopause. Lack of testosterone, a male hormone that women produce in small amounts in their ovaries, is linked to lack of sexual desire. I'm not sure what causes it. I can't find any medical research to explain why this happens, although I firmly believe—as I have said over and over—that poor diet, lack of exercise, and *stress* are major culprits!

Although I haven't met any, some women report a heightened sexual desire and activity before and after menopause. That's not to say there aren't plenty of women who do. The only ones I've met so far have experienced a loss of desire. These are the women whom I hope this book will help. An alternative non-drug approach during the change encourages your body to balance your hormones and heal itself. It should be supported by acupuncture, some form of meditation, herbs, and the natural alternatives that we've discussed so far.

THE LIVER

The liver is a large gland that secretes bile and acts in the formation of blood and in the metabolism of carbohydrates, fat, proteins, and vitamins. The liver is perhaps the most congested of all organs. Too much fat, chemicals, intoxicants, and processed food can all disrupt its intricate biochemical processes. Cigarettes, alcohol, coffee, and refined sugar are destructive to your metabolism as well, and residues from drugs and medication are stored in your liver and other tissues, including your brain. When your liver is healthy, it helps energy to flow through your whole body, but when the liver is impaired it has a trickle-down effect on the rest of the organs of the body. Practitioners of Chinese medicine believe that liver stagnation prevents the flow of energy from the liver to the heart, and can lead to heart disease.

Eating for a Healthy Liver

The liver plays an extremely important role in keeping the body in healthy working order by purifying the blood. If the liver is stagnant, then blood purification may be inadequate, leading to the release of toxins into your body.

In *Healing with Whole Foods,* Paul Pitchford recommends that you eliminate or reduce your consumption of foods that obstruct or damage the liver. These foods include:

- saturated fats, lard, and red meats in large portions
- hydrogenated and poor-quality fats like shortening, margarine, and refined and rancid oils
- excess nuts and seeds
- chemicals in water (drink filtered or bottled water)
- alcohol
- highly processed, refined foods

I never understood why anyone would buy processed foods. It doesn't take very much time to prepare things fresh. The difference in the taste and the nutritional value are so worth the added time (which isn't much, I promise). And if you took the time to read the labels, you would never feed yourself or your family that other stuff. The motto in our house is: If we can't pronounce it, we don't eat it or drink it. Have you ever read the contents on a can of soda?

Of course I may have gone overboard a little bit when I told my kids that hot dogs were made out of ground gorilla lips! Poor things—they went to a friend's house for dinner one evening and came home starving. It seems they served hot dogs for dinner, and my kids wouldn't touch them. I fessed up and told them the truth—that most hot dogs are made with additives, nitrites, food coloring, and preservatives. That worked, too! They do eat hot dogs I buy at the health food store, which are delicious. (You can't go through life without eating hot dogs.) They are made with soy and are called "tofurky" or "smart dogs." I love eating them on a hot, toasted whole-wheat bun with all the trimmings!

Paul Pitchford suggests eating certain foods to help stimulate the liver and prevent stagnation:

- moderately pungent foods, spices, and herbs
- vegetables, including beets, turnips, cauliflower, broccoli, Brussels sprouts, romaine lettuce, asparagus, watercress, mustard greens, and all members of the onion family
- fruits, including strawberries, peaches, and cherries
- chestnuts
- pine nuts
- sprouted grains
- beans
- rye
- quinoa (a grain that can be found in health food stores)

Pitchford also makes the following dietary recommendations:

- Bitter and sour foods are good for the liver. Use unrefined apple cider, brown rice, and rice-wine vinegar.

• Too much extremely pungent food, such as hot peppers, can cause damage to a stagnated liver. Alcohol should also be avoided because it causes cell destruction. If you must drink, do so sparingly.

• Herbs—such as dandelion root (prepare a tea from the root or make a salad out of the leaves), chamomile flowers, bupleurum, which my herbalist has me on, and mild milk thistle seeds—also help reduce liver stagnation.

Milk thistle comes highly recommended by Dr. Andrew Weil in his book *Eight Weeks to Optimum Health*. Here's what he has to say: "[Milk thistle] has great liver protective properties. An extract of the seed, silymarin, enhances metabolism of liver cells and protects them from toxic injury. Conventional medicine has nothing comparable to offer patients with liver problems. And milk thistle products are completely nontoxic and cheap." He recommends milk thistle for all heavy users of alcohol and pharmaceutical drugs that are hard on the liver, including cancer patients undergoing chemotherapy. "It does not interfere with chemotherapy," says Dr. Weil. "When added to a sensible regimen of dietary and lifestyle change, it can return liver function to normal after several months of regular use. If you work with toxic chemicals or feel you have suffered toxic exposures from any source, take milk thistle. It will help your body recover from any harm." Milk thistle can be found in all health-food stores.

Silymarin is found in the seeds of milk thistle. It is

believed that silymarin prompts the manufacture of new, healthy liver cells without encouraging the growth of any malignant liver tissue. Silymarin is thought to serve as an antioxidant, protecting liver cells from damage by free radicals, which are harmful by-products of many bodily processes, including metabolism.

Dr. Weil suggests you rely on standardized extracts of milk thistle. Follow the suggested dosage on the label of the product you buy, or take two tablets or capsules twice a day. He says that you can take milk thistle indefinitely.

People are overmedicating themselves with pain relievers, antibiotics, and pills. Of course, many people need medication, but you should be aware that if you're on any medication for a long period of time, you should eat the proper foods to help your liver eliminate the buildup of toxins in your system.

Some of the recipes I've included in the last chapter contain ingredients that could help your liver:

- Vegetarian Chili
- Tower of Vegetables
- Peach Phyllo Dessert Cups with Strawberry Glaze
- Strawberry Soup

KIDNEYS AND ADRENALS

The kidneys are the organs that filter the blood and excrete the end products of body metabolism in the form of urine, among other duties. The adrenal glands are located directly on top of the kidneys. Paul Pitchford says that they also contribute to the energy, warmth, sexuality, and other attributes of the body.

These two thumb-sized glands produce hormones that allow you to respond to the conditions of your daily life. If the intensity and the frequency of stress in your life become too great, then over time your adrenal glands will begin to become exhausted. Your body will produce many different symptoms in an attempt to get you to pay attention and change some aspects of your life. These are some of the causes of adrenal dysfunction:

- worry
- anger
- guilt
- anxiety
- fear
- depression
- allergies
- surgery
- overwork, physical or mental
- environmental toxins
- chronic pain or illness
- temperature extremes

Along with some sort of meditation or down time every day—you *can* find fifteen to twenty minutes— you should try herbal support.

Siberian ginseng is an excellent remedy for stress-related problems. You can drink it in tea form. I make a pitcherful of iced ginseng tea and keep it in my refrigerator.

Licorice root contains natural plant hormones. You can drink it as a tea or in a tincture. Raspberry tea and blackberry tea are delicious and soothing.

Eat whole, natural, unprocessed foods. Avoid sugar, caffeine, and junk food as much as you can.

Also, for menopausal health you should have your current level of DHEA tested to see if it is in balance. (DHEA stands for dehydroepiandrosterone, a steroid hormone made in your adrenal glands, which your body converts into other hormones.) Some doctors think that DHEA can improve your memory, sex drive, immunity, and sense of vitality and well-being. Your doctor can determine whether or not you should take DHEA and how much you should take.

Being tired and sleep-deprived can add stress and strain your adrenals. Tony and I recently went on a vacation to Hong Kong and Thailand. It was a *very long* trip, and Tony did not feel well when we returned. When he went to see his doctor, he took the adrenal test and found out that he had completely blown them out! It really wasn't the trip that got him. It was me! He's always worried about my comfort because I hate to travel (and I'm very high maintenance), so he tries to do everything he can to make the whole experience more comfortable. Although after our Hong Kong trip he has sworn off traveling with me forever! One Sunday I planned a trip to Santa Barbara, and it took major negotiations just to get him to ride two hours in the car with me!

I always eat wrong when I travel, because there just isn't anything healthy or nourishing to eat. I'm always dumbfounded when I'm at an airport and they offer nothing, and I mean nothing, in the way of a healthy alternative. As I walk and up down the endless corridors of greasy fried foods (which smell so inviting, I might add), I give in and grab something that is totally wrong for me. The fat and salt counts are so high, I blow up two dress sizes right there in the plane during takeoff! I look at everyone around me and they are all angry, tired, and bored. So bored that that we all stuff our faces with foods that just add to more anxiety—especially if you give into the cookies, doughnuts, brownies, and fake frozen yogurt. Who knows what's in that stuff?

THYROID AND PITUITARY

The thyroid gland is located at the base of your neck and wraps around your windpipe. It is shaped like a butterfly. It produces hormones that have a significant impact on brain and body metabolism by regulating the rates at which various cells grow, reproduce, and consume oxygen. Many people, especially middle-aged women, don't produce enough hormones in their thyroid gland. When thyroid function is too low, a woman may experience weight gain, lack of energy, dry skin, brittle nails, and dull hair. When thyroid function is too high, called hyperthyroidism, a woman may experience weight loss, feelings of anxiety and nervousness, inability to relax when tired, and a fast pulse. It is important for you to have your thyroid checked if you experience some of these symptoms.

Thyroid gland malfunction is also believed to cause estrogen imbalances in the body. Imbalances seem to occur during perimenopause because the thyroid gland interacts with the pituitary gland as it attempts to stimulate ovulation. Stress also seems to have a dramatic effect on thyroid function.

The pituitary gland is a bean-shaped organ located at the base of the brain. The hormones secreted by the pituitary stimulate and control the function of many other endocrine (hormone-producing) glands in the body.

You need iodine to make the thyroid hormones that regulate your body's metabolism. A shortage of iodine can lead to hypothyroidism, or underactive thyroid. When that happens, your thyroid gland swells up and forms a lump in your neck called a goiter.

Be sure you speak to your health care adviser before taking any supplements for your thyroid, because thyroid conditions can be tricky to diagnose and treat. For example, too much iodine can throw the thyroid imbalance to another extreme.

If you have hyperthyroidism, eating cabbage,

peaches, rutabagas, soy products, spinach, peanuts, and radishes may help to lower your production of thyroid hormones. But if you have hypothyroidism, it may be best to avoid these foods. Again, talk to your doctor.

7

Help for Alleviating Symptoms of PMS and Menopause—in the Closet!

I'll share with you what works for me. Whenever I feel overwhelmed, and that's every day, there are two things I can always do. One is to go into my closet, close the door, and sit on the floor with my legs crossed. Why I go into the closet is beyond me, but somehow I feel safe there, as if I am in a cocoon. There I take several really deep breaths. I start to pray and give thanks for all the wonderful things in my life. By the time I go through everyone and everything, I'm usually sitting there with tears streaming down my cheeks. Not out of sadness, but relief. The tears are cleansing and seem to release tension. Sometimes I weep and sometimes I don't, but I always get something out of it. When I check my watch, usually ten minutes have gone by, but I feel as if I have taken a sweet nap.

Of course if prayer and closets are not your thing, find whatever place works for you. Just make sure it's somewhere you will not be disturbed for however long you need. Tell whoever is in the house what you're doing and ask that you not be disturbed. Take the phone off the hook.

The second thing I do is tell my family—after homework has been done, dinner has been served, bath time is over, husband has gone through the mail, and we have finished our discussion of the Nei-man Marcus bill that month—that I need fifteen minutes to myself. I wish I could get more, but fifteen seems to be the magic number before someone in my house needs something. I tell everyone that I'm going to be in my bathroom, so they know where I am and why I lock the door and need some privacy. They are very good about it and respect my wishes. However, I feel like a heel when I open the door and the kids are usually sitting right there coloring or reading a book, just waiting for me. It was from those moments that I discovered I could have down time while I enjoy the company of my children.

KIDS ARE PEOPLE, TOO!

Children experience stress as well. There is so much pressure on kids these days. We want them to excel in school, sports, and life. Not to mention all the other extracurricular activities.

My children are up at seven each morning to put in a full day of school, and then have gads of homework to do, sometimes well into the evening. They burn out just like the rest of us. They need to relax.

One evening I asked my girls if they would be interested in doing some stretches and meditation. To my delight, they said yes, and they have been doing it regularly ever since. To start, I have them take a bath using bath salts to relax their bodies. After they're dried off and in a warm pair of jammies, we head to my bedroom where I put on a soothing CD like *The Sea*. After we do some easy stretches and deep breathing, I have them lie on the floor with a pillow cradling their heads. I cover them with a warm blanket or towel. Then we go on our journey. This is their favorite part.

The journey starts with eyes closed. From there we go to faraway places. I guide them along with the power of suggestion. It's fun to make up different places to go. Sometimes we travel by cloud or just fly. By the time we get to our destination, they are asleep or so relaxed I can't move them from the floor. Even if they need to get back to do more homework, they seem to handle it so much better. They always sleep so well and wake up feeling rested and in good spirits.

I try to do this two to three times a week. It makes me feel calm and happy to see how positively it affects them. It also gives me time as a mother just to look at them, touch them, and appreciate what a gift they are and how much I love them! It fills me up and I feel complete. It's a nice way to say good night!

TUB POWER

I'm a big believer in the power of the tub. I love to soak in a steaming bath with bath oils or salts that have a heavenly aroma. As you inhale, the aroma takes over your senses and brings a welcome sense of relief.

If bath oils are not in your budget, you can make your own. Simply buy a large bottle of mineral oil. It's priced very reasonably. Take any size glass jar and fill it to almost the top. To make it look pretty, you can cut the tops off dried flowers and drop them in. Add whatever scent you like. You can usually buy beautiful scents at your arts and crafts stores. They come in a variety of soothing aromas.

My favorites are jasmine and rose. You can mix whatever you like to make a calming aroma. After you fill your glass jar, cover it with a lid or cork to keep it fresh. It should stay fresh for about a month. When you are ready to bathe, pour about a capful under comfortably hot running water. Fill your tub to the top and sink right in, taking time to feel your body relax as you slide to the bottom. Place a towel underneath your head. At this point, you can do anything you want—read a book, listen to music, or simply stare at the ceiling. When you have completed your quiet time, gently dry off and rub on your favorite body lotion. You are now ready to face the rest of your day or evening with a new attitude.

IDEAS TO HELP YOU MOVE

The E word—exercise! I guess there's just no way around it. If you want to remain in good working order, you need to move your parts.

I go in spurts. I can go for months exercising three to four times a week and months of just being sedentary. When I do exercise, I feel so much better. My skin improves, my appetite decreases, I walk with so much more confidence, my sex life improves, and my pants zip up!

Exercise is even more crucial for woman who suffer from PMS or who are going through menopause.

After menopause, women are more susceptible to heart disease. Your cholesterol rises and you lose bone mass. Exercise plays a major part in staying healthy! The most important thing to remember is that you need to do at least thirty to forty minutes of cardiovascular exercise three to four times a week. You will reap many benefits from it and feel both mentally and physically fit. Of course, if you do not exercise regularly, you should consult with a doctor before starting an exercise program. When your body is going through so much, exercise is your secret weapon!

Walking

What makes the biggest difference when I walk is putting a great CD or tape in my Walkman that makes me want to move to the beat. There are great tapes available today. Go to the section of a music store where the exercise tapes are and find some contemporary music with a disco or salsa beat. Pick out music you can just rock to!

Also, pick up some videotapes on aerobics you can do in your home. And buy a tape on stepping. Even if you do not have step equipment in your home, watch it anyway. It will give you great ideas when you are out for a walk. If you walk on the street, you can use the curb to do some of the step exercises. Your neighbors might think you're a little odd, but who cares?

Or you can use a treadmill. If you don't have one, you can power walk. That is walking at a fast clip with your arms swinging back and forth over your waist. The arms swinging will help elevate your heart rate.

You can go to your local high school or college campus and walk around the track. There are usually bleachers around the track area as well. I go to our local college campus and use the track and the stairs. There are fifteen sets of fifty-one steps. When I first started, I would walk around the track twice to warm up, and then do two sets of stairs. The next time three, then four, and I kept on adding until I could do all fifteen sets, up and down. I do them at a pace that is right for me. It usually takes me forty minutes. I get the benefit of aerobics and toning. There is nothing better for your buns!

If you have steps in your home, use them. Go up and down the steps at whatever pace you can for at least twenty minutes.

Swimming

Swimming is probably the best form of exercise because it doesn't put strain on your body. If you don't have access to a pool, you can go to your local YMCA.

You can purchase a set of special equipment at your local sports store with a vest that will keep you afloat in the water. You can actually jog back and forth in the pool with no impact on your bones at all. I place the vest around my upper body, and it holds me upright. The whole set comes with water exercise dumbbells for the upper body and low-impact footwear to strengthen leg muscles. As an alternative it's great, because you can get bored doing the same exercise over and over again. Using this equipment is really fun and you can actually feel the benefit of the exercise without the strain, because your body is weightless in the water. Thirty to forty-five minutes will be enough.

Bicycling

Bicycle, either indoors on a stationary bike or outdoors, thirty to forty minutes several times a week.

Weights

No matter what other exercise you do, it's important to begin exercising with weights. You don't have to spend hours in the gym pumping iron. You only need to use light weights three to four times a week to strengthen your arms, chest, and legs. Weight-bearing exercise is especially crucial for women who are going through menopause or have reached menopause, because it helps build bone mass.

You don't have to do all these exercises together. You can do your cardiovascular workout one day and your weights the next. I can feel the difference! My body is so much stronger.

Make sure you ask your doctor for a bone density test so you can monitor and actually do something about bone loss. Remember, it's up to you!

HOW AM I DOING?

The road to feeling better has been an adventure, to say the least. In the process I've learned a lot about myself and how much my husband really loves me! In all, it took about eight years. Eight years of struggling with personality and mood swings that were very destructive. I compromised my marriage, co-workers, and friends many times because I didn't understand what was going on with my body. There does come a time when you say to yourself, *Enough!*

Lucky for me I came out the other end still surrounded by the people I love, the people who mean the most to me.

Eight years is a very long time. I just didn't want to accept the fact that what I was eating—because I really *love* to eat—and my lack of discipline in exercising were keeping me from feeling good! I would exercise or eat healthily for about a week or two, then give up, because *it takes work!*

Now I have incorporated soy and my new way of eating into my everyday life. Since I've done so, I have noticed a huge difference in the way I feel and move. I'm eating more fruits and vegetables, and they in turn keep life's energy flow in working order.

I am diligent in sticking to my exercise regime.

I don't know what came over me one day. My husband and I decided to have lunch together. Instead of driving into Beverly Hills, approximately four miles from where we live, we walked. We had a lovely lunch together then headed home, four miles back. I was so proud of our accomplishment that I now do this at least once a week. It's done so much for me mentally. It's made me feel good about myself, and I can see the difference in my hair, my skin, and the firmness of my body! There is a huge difference in my stamina, not to mention my legs and thighs. Now when Tony reaches for me he's not feeling flabby thighs and a soft stomach.

My sex drive has returned! Okay, not the way it was in the beginning—but my god, at least I'm feeling horny again! I actually initiate sex. *Shock!* The vitamins have kicked in, the healthy eating is working, and the cream gives me that extra boost I need!

My PMS is under control. My terrible mood swings have disappeared. I no longer become despondent, and my aggressive habits have subsided to where I am not obnoxious. All is well at home, and I'm feeling wonderful!

The most important thing I do for myself—it makes a world of difference—is to drink twelve eight-ounce glasses of water every day. It flushes everything out, and keeps your skin hydrated and looking younger. It is, in my opinion, the fountain of youth!

I'm only human. I still reach for chocolate or want ice cream or a burger, but I don't beat myself up over it. Besides, I really don't feel so great afterward, so I'm more than ready to go back to healthy eating habits again.

8

Eating for a Healthier You

I have compiled some recipes that are easy to prepare, rich in natural plant estrogens, and delicious. Your family will enjoy them, and at the same
time they will be introduced to a healthier way of
eating. However, the most important message that I
want to give you is the necessity of including soy
products in your diet. They're my secret weapon.

THE JOY OF SOY

I became interested in soy because of all the health
benefits I learned they supply. The little soybean is
jam-packed with a protein and hormonelike substance called isoflavones. They have been known to
reduce cholesterol, build bone mass, and help alleviate

hot flashes. There is also a possible reduction in the risk of prostate and breast cancers.

When I mention that I'm eating soy products, most people cringe and make a face. The thought of eating tofu and drinking soy milk is not appealing to some people. I must admit it wasn't to me, either, in the beginning. Eating tofu was like eating a sponge. It had no flavor whatsoever, and a strange texture. But it's lucky that tofu doesn't have a flavor, since it will take on whatever flavor you give it.

Soy products come in a variety of different forms. There are soy wieners, roasted soy nuts (one of my favorite snacks), chocolate-coated bars, and something I'm absolutely addicted to—miso.

Miso is a fermented soybean paste. I use it as a soup base and have it for breakfast with cut-up tofu. It's steaming hot and sends me off to start my day with plenty of protein and energy. I also use it as a snack when I'm dragging or simply hungry. Sometimes I add steamed rice and have a bowl for lunch or dinner. It is rich in plant estrogens.

Fresh soybeans, called edamame, are great to snack on as well. They come frozen, and you can usually find them in health-food stores, although I notice that supermarkets are starting to carry them, too. They consist of pods containing the soy beans, and you steam them. You break open the pods and enjoy a deliciously protein-packed snack. I *love* them, and so do my kids.

Please don't let the idea of eating soy products

deter you from making this ever-so-important change in your diet. I have included recipes in this book that I have worked on diligently, testing them on my family and friends. I have come away time and time again with glowing reports of how much they enjoyed the meals and how absolutely delicious everything was.

Following are some recipes that are easy to prepare, rich in natural plant estrogens and/or low in fat, and delicious.

Bon Appetit!

✑ BREAKFAST TREATS

Bran Muffins
Whole Wheat Blueberry Pancakes
Egg White Omelet
Potato and Onion Frittata

✑ SALADS, DRESSINGS, AND SALSAS

Tower of Veggies
Raspberry Dijon Dressing
Springtime Raspberry Dressing
Wonderful Tofu Caesar Dressing
Oriental Dressing
Creamy Italian Dressing
Creamy Yogurt Dressing
Nonfat Thousand Island Dressing
Tomato Salsa
Pineapple-Mango Salsa
Papaya or Mango Salsa

✑ SOUPS

Miso Soup
Potato and Leek Soup
Curried Carrot Soup
Creamy Corn Soup
Ginger Garlic Soup
Pasta Fagioli Soup
Tomato, Pasta, and White Bean Soup
Vegetarian Chili

SANDWICHES

Terrific Tofu "Egg" Salad Sandwiches
Grilled Cheese and Tomato Sandwich
Caraway Tuna Salad Sandwiches
Chinese Chicken Wrap
Club Sandwich

PASTAS

Lasagna with Six Vegetables
Greek Pasta with Tomatoes and Beans
Farfalle with No-Cook Fresh Tomato Sauce
Fusilli with Smoked Salmon and Caviar

VEGETABLES

Spaghetti Squash with Fresh Tomato Sauce
Crusty Potato Fillets
Bok Choy
Candied Carrots

MAIN DISHES

Mexican Black Bean Burger
Low-Fat Crepes with Ratatouille Filling
Thai Sweet-and-Sour Prawns
Oriental Roasted Salmon
Sea Bass with Lemon and Capers
Raspberry-Glazed Chicken
Cornmeal-Crusted Chicken
Thai Minced Chicken in Lettuce Leaves
Good-for-You Cheeseburgers with Unfried Potatoes

∽ ANYTIME SNACKS AND SMOOTHIES

Soybean Hummus
Low-Fat Egg Rolls
Snack Foods
Strawberry-Banana Tofu Smoothie
Orange Velvet Deluxe
Banana Chocolate Soyprise
Perfect Piña Colada
Strawberry Soup

∽ DESSERTS

Banana Split
Soy-Enriched Creamy Rice Pudding
Apple Phyllo
Peach Phyllo Dessert Cups
Chocolate Brownies

BREAKFAST TREATS

Bran Muffins

16 MUFFINS

Cooking spray
1 ½ cups unprocessed wheat bran
1 cup whole wheat flour
1 tablespoon grated orange peel
1 teaspoon baking soda
¼ teaspoon salt
1 ½ cups low-fat buttermilk
3 tablespoons dark molasses
1 large egg, lightly beaten
2 tablespoons canola oil
½ cup raisins

Preheat oven to 375°F. Spray 16 muffin cups with cooking spray. In a large bowl, stir together the wheat bran, flour, orange peel, baking soda, and salt. In a second bowl, whisk together the buttermilk, molasses, egg, and oil. Add liquid ingredients to dry ingredients and stir just until dry ingredients are moistened. Do not overmix. Fold in raisins.

Fill muffin pans ¾ full. Bake for 14 to 16 minutes or until a wooden pick inserted in the center comes out clean. Turn out onto a cooling rack; serve warm with a tablespoon of orange marmalade, or peach or cherry preserves.

Whole Wheat Blueberry Pancakes

12 PANCAKES

 2 cups whole wheat flour
 2 teaspoons baking powder
 1/2 teaspoon baking soda
 1/4 teaspoon salt
 2 cups low-fat buttermilk
 1 tablespoon honey
 2 teaspoons canola oil
 2 teaspoons grated lemon peel
 1 teaspoon vanilla
 1 egg, slightly beaten
 2 egg whites
 1 cup blueberries
 Additional canola oil or cooking spray
 Maple syrup and fresh fruit slices, as desired

In a large bowl, sift together the dry ingredients. In another bowl, whisk together the buttermilk, honey, oil, lemon peel, and vanilla. Whisk in the 1 egg.

In a small bowl, beat the egg whites with an electric mixer on high speed until stiff peaks form. Stir the honey mixture into the flour mixture just until blended (mixture may be slightly lumpy). With a rubber spatula, fold egg whites gently into batter until no traces of white remain (do not stir). Carefully fold in blueberries.

With a little canola oil on paper toweling, or cooking spray, coat the surface of a griddle or an iron skillet. Heat griddle or skillet over medium heat. Ladle batter onto griddle in 5- or 6-inch circles. Cook 2 to 3 minutes, until pancakes look bubbly on the top; turn and cook a few minutes more until done.

Transfer pancakes to a warm platter. Serve with genuine maple syrup and fresh fruit.

Egg White Omelet

1 SERVING

Three egg whites
Cooking spray
One scallion, chopped
$1/4$ cup red pepper, diced
$1/2$ cup mushrooms (I prefer shiitake for richer flavor)
(optional)
$1/4$ teaspoon dried basil
$1/8$ teaspoon salt
$1/8$ teaspoon pepper

In a small mixing bowl, whisk egg whites just until they become frothy. Mix in the basil, salt, and pepper.

Liberally spray a small skillet with vegetable cooking spray and sauté vegetables over medium-high heat until tender.

Pour egg mixture over vegetables. As the eggs start to set, use a spatula to lift edge of eggs and turn them over. As soon as all the mixture has set, remove pan from heat and fold the omelet in half. Serve immediately.

Spoon some of your favorite salsa on top!

Potato and Onion Frittata

4 TO 6 SERVINGS

Cooking spray
1 to 2 tablespoons olive oil
8 small new potatoes, sliced ⅛-inch thick
1 ½ cups sliced onion
2 shallots, minced
2 cloves garlic, minced
4 egg whites
2 large eggs
1 tablespoon chopped fresh basil
1 tablespoon chopped Italian parsley
¼ teaspoon each salt and pepper
1 ounce (¼ cup) crumbled feta cheese

Spray a heavy ovenproof skillet with cooking spray. Add oil and heat over medium-high heat. Sauté the potatoes, onions, shallots, and garlic for 5 minutes, stirring frequently. Reduce heat; cover and cook 3 to 5 minutes more until the potatoes are tender, stirring frequently.

Meanwhile, whisk together in a bowl the egg whites, eggs, basil, parsley, salt, and pepper. Spread the vegetables evenly in the pan; pour egg mixture over vegetables. Sprinkle feta cheese evenly over the top. Transfer the pan to the oven; bake for 8 to 10 minutes more, or until a knife inserted just off-center comes out clean.

Let stand for 2 minutes and cut into wedges. Serve with salsa, if desired. Refrigerate any leftovers.

SALADS, DRESSINGS, AND SALSAS

Tower of Veggies

8 SERVINGS

2 cups cooked couscous
2 tablespoons fresh lemon juice
2 tablespoons chopped parsley
1 tablespoon olive oil
1 cup sliced cucumber
¼ cup seasoned rice vinegar
1 empty, clean soup can with both ends removed
2 cups of baby salad greens or mixed salad greens, torn
Raspberry Dijon Dressing (p. 107)
1 cup chopped celery
1 cup roasted red bell peppers, skinned, seeded, well-
    drained, and chopped
4 ounces (1 cup) crumbled feta cheese or goat cheese
1 cup diced tomatoes
Chopped parsley and chopped fresh basil for garnish
    (optional)

In a medium bowl, stir together the couscous, lemon
juice, parsley, and oil. Set aside. In another bowl, toss
the cucumbers with the vinegar. Set aside. In another
bowl, toss the salad greens with the Raspberry Dijon
Dressing.

To assemble each individual salad, use the empty

soup can to mold each "tower." Place the soup can upright on a salad plate. Insert ¼ cup of the greens on the bottom, inside the can. Press down with fingers. Spoon ¼ cup of the couscous mixture over lettuce, pressing down with the back of a spoon. Layer 2 tablespoons each of the celery, peppers, cheese, tomatoes, and cucumber mixture on top. Press down to condense the stack inside the can. Carefully lift the can upwards. You should have a beautifully presented tower of veggies. Top with chopped parsley and basil. I love toasted olive bread or rosemary bread with this.

Raspberry Dijon Dressing

²/₃ CUP

  ½ cup raspberry vinegar
  2 tablespoons seasoned rice vinegar
  1 tablespoon Dijon mustard
  ¼ teaspoon sugar

In a medium glass bowl, whisk together all ingredients. Drizzle over salad and toss.

Springtime Raspberry Dressing

1 1/4 CUPS

> 1/2 cup extra virgin olive oil
> 2 tablespoons Dijon mustard
> 1/2 cup raspberry vinegar
> 2 tablespoons seasoned rice vinegar
> I tablespoon balsamic vinegar
> 1/4 teaspoon sugar
> I clove garlic, crushed

In a glass bowl, whisk together the olive oil and mustard. Add vinegars and sugar. Place in a glass jar, add the garlic, and refrigerate. Remove the garlic after one hour, to prevent possible growth of bacteria. Dressing (with garlic removed) will keep for up to a week if refrigerated.

Wonderful Tofu Caesar Dressing

1 CUP

4 ounces (½ cup) soft tofu, drained
⅓ cup olive oil (extra virgin recommended)
2 tablespoons Dijon or yellow mustard
1 clove garlic, quartered
1 to 2 anchovy fillets, rinsed
2 teaspoons Worcestershire sauce
Juice of 1 lemon (3 tablespoons)

In a blender or food processor, place all ingredients; cover and blend until smooth. Refrigerate any leftovers. Store dressing in refrigerator for up to 3 days.

Oriental Dressing

1 CUP

> ½ cup seasoned rice vinegar
> ⅓ cup olive oil (extra virgin recommended)
> 2 tablespoons lemon juice
> Juice of ½ lime (1 tablespoon)
> ½ teaspoon sesame oil

In a small bowl, whisk together all ingredients until well blended. To eliminate the fat calories, omit the oil.

Creamy Italian Dressing

1 CUP

4 ounces (½ cup) soft tofu, drained
⅓ cup olive oil (extra virgin recommended)
2 tablespoons red wine vinegar
1 tablespoon balsamic vinegar
1 tablespoon Dijon mustard
1 teaspoon dried oregano, crushed
1 teaspoon dried basil, crushed
¼ teaspoon salt
¼ teaspoon pepper
¼ teaspoon sugar
1 small clove garlic, minced

Place all ingredients in blender container or food processor bowl. Cover and blend until smooth. Dressing will last several days if refrigerated.

Creamy Yogurt Dressing

1 1/3 CUPS

- 2 cups plain yogurt
- Juice of 1 lemon (3 tablespoons)
- 1 tablespoon dried oregano, crushed
- 1 tablespoon dried basil, crushed
- 1 tablespoon dillweed, crushed
- 1/2 teaspoon salt
- 1/2 teaspoon pepper (optional)
- Vegetable dippers, such as sliced cucumbers, baby carrots, broccoli florets, zucchini sticks, or jicama sticks

Line a medium strainer with a coffee filter; place it over a small bowl. Add yogurt, cover with plastic wrap, and allow yogurt to drain for 2 hours. It will resemble a soft cheese. Discard the drained liquid.

In a medium bowl whisk together the drained yogurt and remaining ingredients, except vegetables. My kids love to eat this dip on raw vegetables.

Nonfat Thousand Island Dressing

$^3/_4$ CUP

- $^1/_2$ cup nonfat mayonnaise
- $^1/_4$ cup catsup
- 1 tablespoon minced sweet pickle, or drained pickle relish
- $^1/_2$ to 1 teaspoon bottled hot pepper sauce

In a small bowl stir together all ingredients until well blended. Cover and store in refrigerator for up to a week.

Tomato Salsa

5 1/2 CUPS

  8 Roma or 4 medium tomatoes, seeded and chopped
      (2 cups)
  1/2 cup chopped red onion
  1/2 cup chopped yellow onion
  1/4 cup chopped cilantro or parsley
  1 jalapeño pepper, minced
  Juice of 1 lemon (3 tablespoons)
  Juice of 2 limes (1/4 cup)
  1 teaspoon dried red pepper flakes, crushed (optional)
  1/2 teaspoon salt

In a medium bowl, combine all ingredients. Cover
and let stand, or chill, for at least 30 minutes to blend
flavors. Keeps for several days. Recipe can be halved.

Pineapple-Mango Salsa

6 CUPS

2 cups chopped fresh pineapple
2 mangoes, peeled and chopped
1 small cucumber, peeled, seeded, and diced
$\frac{1}{2}$ cup chopped red onion
$\frac{1}{3}$ cup chopped cilantro
$\frac{1}{3}$ cup fresh lime juice
$\frac{1}{4}$ chopped red bell pepper
3 scallions, thinly sliced
1 jalapeño pepper, minced (optional)
$\frac{1}{4}$ teaspoon salt

In a large bowl, combine all ingredients. Cover and chill for at least 30 minutes to blend flavors. Keeps for several days. Recipe can be halved.

Serve this salsa on seafood, grilled chicken, or burritos.

Papaya or Mango Salsa

4 CUPS

> 2 papayas or mangoes, peeled, seeded, and chopped
> 1 small cucumber, peeled, seeded, and chopped
> 4 scallions, thinly sliced
> 2 teaspoons chopped cilantro or parsley
> 1/3 cup fresh lime juice
> 2 tablespoons low-sodium soy sauce

In a medium nonmetal bowl, combine all ingredients. Cover and refrigerate at least 1 hour to blend flavors. Keeps for 3 days.

Serve this salsa on seafood or grilled chicken.

Soups

Miso Soup

1 SERVING

I tablespoon miso paste
I cup boiling water
½ scallion, minced
½ teaspoon chopped cilantro

Stir the miso paste into the boiling water; reduce heat
and simmer for 1 minute. Pour into a heated bowl
and sprinkle with scallions and cilantro.

You can find miso with Asian ingredients in the
dairy case. I also like to add rice, or some cut-up
chicken pieces, or both, with the scallions and cilantro.

Potato and Leek Soup

8 SERVINGS

> 2 tablespoons olive oil
> 1 cup finely chopped yellow onion
> 2 leeks, chopped (white part only)
> 5 cups peeled, diced Idaho potatoes
> 4 cups chicken or vegetable stock or broth
> Corn cut from 2 fresh cobs, or 1 15-ounce can niblet
>   corn, drained
> 8 ounces (1 cup) soft tofu, drained and cut up
> 8-ounce package nonfat cream cheese
> Salt and pepper to taste
> Chopped dill for garnish (optional)

In a Dutch oven or stockpot heat the olive oil. Add the chopped onion and leeks and sauté for 2 minutes. Stir in potatoes and cook 5 minutes, stirring frequently. Add the stock and the corn; bring mixture to boiling. Reduce heat and simmer about 15 minutes, or until potatoes are tender.

In a blender or food processor, puree the soup in batches with the tofu and cream cheese until smooth. Add 1 cup more chicken stock or broth if you like a thinner consistency. Return soup to pot; season to taste with salt and pepper. Heat through, but do not boil. Serve piping hot in preheated bowls. Or chill the soup thoroughly, and serve it in bowls you have placed in the freezer for 5 minutes. Garnish with dill if desired.

Curried Carrot Soup

6 SERVINGS

  2 tablespoons olive oil
  1 cup chopped yellow onion
  1 leek, chopped (white part only)
  4 cups chopped carrots
  4 cups chicken or vegetable stock or broth
  1 teaspoon curry powder
  4 ounces (½ cup) soft tofu, drained
  4 ounces (½ cup) nonfat cream cheese
  1 teaspoon salt
  Chopped chives and nonfat dairy sour cream for
     garnish

In a Dutch oven or stockpot, heat the olive oil. Add the onions and chopped leek. Sauté for 2 minutes. Add the chopped carrots and sauté for 5 minutes, stirring frequently. Add the stock and curry; bring mixture to boiling. Reduce heat and simmer, partially covered, for about 10 to 15 minutes or until carrots are tender.

In a blender or food processor, puree the soup in batches with the tofu and cream cheese until smooth. Return soup to the pot; stir in salt. Serve soup in hot bowls, garnished with chives and a dollop of sour cream. Or chill the soup thoroughly and serve cold, garnished the same way, for an excellent summer meal. Serve with a nice big salad.

If you don't like curry, just eliminate it from the recipe. The soup still tastes great.

Creamy Corn Soup

4 TO 6 SERVINGS

    Corn cut from 4 fresh cobs, or 2 15-ounce cans niblet
        corn, drained
    Cooking spray
    1 tablespoon olive oil
    2 stalks celery, chopped
    1 yellow onion, quartered
    1/2 jalapeño pepper (optional)
    6 cups chicken stock or broth
    4 ounces (1/2 cup) soft tofu, drained
    4 ounces (1/2 cup) nonfat cream cheese
    1/4 teaspoon salt
    Chopped chives for garnish (optional)

Reserve 1/2 cup of the corn for garnish. Spray a 3-quart saucepan with cooking spray; add oil and heat to medium-high. Sauté the remaining corn with celery, onion, and jalapeño, if desired, for 5 minutes or until crisp-tender.

Stir in chicken stock and bring mixture to boiling. Reduce heat and simmer, uncovered, for 40 minutes. Remove from heat and cool slightly.

In a blender or food processor, puree the soup in batches, adding tofu and cream cheese to the last batch to be pureed. Return to saucepan; stir in reserved corn and salt. Heat through, if necessary. Serve hot or chilled, garnished with chives if desired.

Ginger Garlic Soup

8 TO 10 SERVINGS

Carcass of 1 or 2 baked or roasted chickens, or 1
   whole roasting chicken, uncooked
4 celery stalks with the leaves, chopped
2 cups chopped carrots
1 medium onion, thinly sliced
6 slices peeled fresh gingerroot
6 cloves garlic
1 bunch cilantro leaves
Water (up to 2 quarts, or 8 cups)
4 ounces vermicelli or spaghetti noodles, cooked,
   drained, and cut into bite-sized pieces
1 cup cooked shredded chicken
$\frac{1}{2}$ cup julienne-sliced carrots
$\frac{1}{2}$ cup bean sprouts
$\frac{1}{2}$ cup snow peas (halve any large peas)
$\frac{1}{2}$ cup chopped scallions
4 ounces vermicelli or spaghettini noodles, cooked,
   drained and cut into bite-sized pieces
Salt and pepper to taste

I always save the bones from roasted chickens to
make this basic broth. It is delicious and hearty, and
I use it to flavor a lot of my dishes. You can make the
same recipe with a raw chicken. It will be lighter but
still lovely.

In a large stockpot place the chicken bones or the
washed whole chicken with giblets removed, celery,
carrots, onion, gingerroot, garlic, and cilantro with
enough water to cover. Bring mixture to boiling. Reduce heat and simmer, uncovered, one hour. Strain
and skim off fat. (Or, cool strained broth and refriger-

ate, covered, overnight. Remove the hardened layer of fat from the broth and reheat strained broth in the stockpot.)

Return the strained broth to the stockpot and heat through. Add the cooked noodles and season to taste with salt and pepper. Ladle hot soup into heated bowls and float in each bowl some of the diced chicken, several strands of the julienne carrots, some bean sprouts, two or three snow peas, a sprinkle of scallions, and some chopped cilantro.

Pasta Fagioli Soup

10 SERVINGS

2 teaspoons olive oil
1 medium onion, finely chopped
3 scallions, finely chopped
8 cloves garlic, minced
1 teaspoon ground sage
1 tablespoon tomato paste
4 cups chicken or vegetable stock or broth
2 15-ounce cans cannellini or navy beans, drained
8 ounces (1 cup) soft tofu, drained and cut up
8 ounces miniature bow tie or small shell pasta,
    cooked, drained, and set aside
1 teaspoon salt
Balsamic vinegar as needed (optional)
Chopped parsley and basil for garnish

In a Dutch oven or large soup pot, heat the olive oil. Add the onion, scallions, garlic, and sage; sauté about 3 minutes or until tender. Add tomato paste; stir constantly for 1 minute. Add stock and drained beans; bring mixture to boiling. Reduce heat and simmer for 15 minutes to blend flavors. Add tofu. Let cool slightly.

In a blender or food processor, puree the soup in batches until smooth. Return soup to the pot. Stir in the cooked, drained pasta and salt. Heat through

To serve, ladle into hot bowls, then drizzle about 1 tablespoon of balsamic vinegar over the top, if desired. Sprinkle with fresh chopped parsley and basil. This soup also freezes well.

Tomato, Pasta, and White Bean Soup

12 SERVINGS

1 cup dried (or 2 15-ounce cans) navy beans, rinsed
and drained
Water for cooking dried beans
1/4 cup olive oil
1 medium onion, chopped
4 cloves garlic, minced
2 teaspoons dried sage, crushed
1 teaspoon dried oregano, crushed
1 1/2 quarts (6 cups) fat-free chicken stock or broth (If
you use canned broth, look for low sodium and no
MSG.)
1 quart water
1 1/2 cups skinned, seeded, chopped tomatoes, or 1 15-
ounce can diced tomatoes, undrained
2 tablespoons chopped fresh chives
8 ounces elbow macaroni or small shell pasta
Chopped fresh parsley for garnish

If using the dry beans, combine the beans and 6 cups
cold water in a saucepan. Bring to boiling; reduce
heat. Simmer 2 minutes. Remove from heat; cover
and let stand one hour. (Or, omit simmering; soak
beans in cold water overnight in a covered pan.)
Drain and rinse the beans and combine in the same
pan with 6 cups fresh water. Bring to boiling; reduce
heat. Cover and simmer for 1 to 1 1/2 hours. Drain
well.

In a 5-quart stockpot, heat the oil. Sauté the onion
with garlic, sage, and oregano until vegetables are
soft and golden. Stir in chicken stock, water, tomatoes, chives, and cooked beans. Bring mixture to boil-

ing; reduce heat. Simmer, uncovered, for 30 minutes to blend flavors. Stir in dried pasta and cook 10 minutes longer or until pasta in done. Serve immediately in bowls garnished with chopped fresh parsley.

Vegetarian Chili

12 TO 14 SERVINGS

1/3 cup olive oil
2 large onions, halved and thinly sliced
4 cloves garlic, minced
2 15-ounce cans kidney beans, rinsed and drained
2 cups thinly sliced mushrooms
4 stalks celery, chopped
3 cups chopped carrots
2 zucchini, cut into bite-sized pieces
1 29-ounce can tomato puree
1 29-ounce can diced tomatoes with juice
2 tablespoons chili powder
1 teaspoon cumin
1 teaspoon coriander
4 ounces (1/2 cup) firm tofu, drained and chopped
Salt and pepper to taste
Nonfat dairy sour cream, chopped red or yellow
    onions, sliced scallions, low-fat shredded cheddar
    or Monterey jack cheese, and cilantro for garnishes
    (optional)

In a 5-quart stockpot, heat the olive oil over medium-high heat. Sauté the onion and garlic until golden. Stir in the drained beans, mushrooms, celery, carrots, and zucchini; sauté for 5 minutes. Stir in tomato puree, tomatoes, chili powder, cumin, and coriander.

Bring mixture to boiling; reduce heat. Simmer, covered, for 45 minutes to blend flavors. Uncover and stir in tofu; cook 15 minutes more, or until desired consistency is reached. Season to taste with salt and pepper. Serve chili in bowls topped with desired garnishes.

SANDWICHES

Terrific Tofu "Egg" Salad Sandwiches

2 CUPS

8 ounces (1 cup) extrafirm tofu, drained
1/3 cup nonfat or low-fat mayonnaise
1 tablespoon Dijon or yellow mustard
2 stalks celery, finely chopped
2 scallions, thinly sliced
1 kosher dill pickle, finely chopped
2 tablespoons minced parsley
1/2 teaspoon curry powder (optional)

Chop tofu into small pieces that resemble chopped eggs. In a medium bowl stir tofu together with remaining ingredients until well combined. Cover and chill for about 1 hour. Serve on whole wheat, rye, or seven-grain bread.

I like to make the sandwiches with toasted bread, a little extra Dijon mustard, a slice of tomato, and alfalfa sprouts. I also enjoy it on a bed of baby greens and stuffed into a vine-ripened tomato. Sprinkle a little fresh basil on top.

If you do not want to eat the tofu, you can still make the egg salad using only hard boiled egg whites. Boil the eggs until hard. Peel, cut in half, and remove the yolk. Cut the egg whites into pieces and add the remaining ingredients.

Grilled Cheese and Tomato Sandwich

1 SERVING

> 1 slice seven-grain, whole wheat, or rye bread
> Stone-ground or Dijon mustard
> 1 or 2 slices tomato
> 1 ounce (1/4 cup) shredded cheese, such as Monterey
> jack, sharp cheddar, Swiss, gouda, or Gruyère

Preheat the broiler. On a baking sheet toast bread until light golden brown on both sides. Spread mustard over bread. Top with tomato slice(s) and sprinkled cheese. Place under broiler for 2 minutes, or until cheese melts and begins to bubble. Cut into halves or quarters and serve with a light salad or cut-up vegetables.

Caraway Tuna Salad Sandwiches

3 CUPS

12-ounce can water-packed tuna, well-drained
1/2 cup nonfat or low-fat mayonnaise
2 stalks celery, finely chopped
3 scallions, thinly sliced
2 tablespoons chopped fresh basil, or 2 teaspoons
    dried basil, crushed
2 tablespoons minced kosher dill pickle, or 1
    tablespoon pickle relish
2 tablespoons lemon juice
2 teaspoons caraway seeds

Transfer tuna to a medium bowl; break into flakes with a fork. Stir in remaining ingredients until well combined.

Serve on rye, wheat, or seven-grain bread, with lettuce, tomatoes, sprouts, and Dijon mustard. For a tuna salad plate, serve on a bed of fresh baby greens with a light vinaigrette. During the summer I like to stuff a vine-ripened tomato with this salad and garnish it with fresh basil. I store cans of tuna in the refrigerator to keep them chilled for this salad.

Chinese Chicken Wrap

7 SERVINGS

    1 cup finely shredded romaine lettuce
    1 cup shredded carrot
    1 small cucumber, peeled, seeded, and chopped
    2 scallions, thinly sliced
    1/2 head red cabbage, shredded (3 cups)
    1 boned, skinned, cooked chicken breast, chopped
        (3/4 cup)
    1/4 cup chopped cilantro
    1 tablespoon toasted sesame seeds
    1/2 cup Oriental Dressing, page 110
    7 burrito-size, low-fat flour tortillas
    7 slices avocado

In a medium bowl, stir together vegetables with chicken, cilantro, and sesame seeds. Drizzle with Oriental Dressing to moisten the mixture.

To assemble wraps, place each tortilla on a flat work surface and spoon a scant 1 cup of the filling on the lower half of the tortilla. Add a slice of avocado. Roll the bottom, then the top, of the tortilla over filling to make a cylinder, then tuck the sides under and place seam-side down on a plate. Slice each roll diagonally across the middle.

Club Sandwich

1 SERVING

> 3 slices whole wheat or seven-grain bread, toasted or
>   untoasted
> 1 tablespoon Dijon mustard
> 1 small half chicken breast, sliced thin (optional)
> 1 or 2 pieces of romaine or Bibb lettuce
> 2 slices tomato
> 1 tablespoon Soybean Hummus, page 155
> 8 1/8-inch-thick slices cucumber
> 1/4 cup alfalfa or broccoli sprouts
> 1 tablespoon nonfat mayonnaise

Spread the mustard on one slice of the bread. Add the
chicken, lettuce, and tomato. Top with the second
slice of bread. On top of that piece of bread spread the
hummus. Add the cucumber, avocado, and sprouts.
Spread the third slice of bread with the mayonnaise
and place it on top of the sandwich. Cut the sandwich into quarters.

Serve with baked tortilla chips, nonfat sourdough
pretzels, or nonfat potato chips.

PASTAS

Lasagna with Six Vegetables

12 SERVINGS

Sauce:
2 tablespoons olive oil
2 medium carrots, finely chopped (1½ cups)
2 celery stalks, finely chopped
1 cup finely chopped yellow onion
2 scallions, finely chopped
29-ounce can, plus 16-ounce can, tomato puree
    or tomato sauce

Lasagna:
12 lasagna noodles
15-ounce package low-fat ricotta cheese
14-ounce package soft tofu, drained
1 pound fresh spinach leaves, steamed, squeezed
    dry, and chopped; or 10-ounce package frozen
    chopped spinach, thawed and squeezed dry
1 teaspoon ground nutmeg
½ teaspoon salt
2 tablespoons butter
2 tablespoons all-purpose flour
1 cup light or low-fat soy milk
Cooking spray
1 cup freshly grated Parmesan cheese
Fresh basil leaves for garnish

For the sauce, heat the olive oil in a 3-quart saucepan. Add the carrots, celery, onion, and scallions. Sauté vegetables about 5 minutes or until tender. Stir in tomato puree or sauce and bring mixture to boiling. Reduce heat and simmer, partially covered, for 20 minutes.

Meanwhile, cook the noodles according to package directions. Drain and rinse in cool water. Lay noodles flat on a dry towel. In a large bowl, stir together the ricotta cheese, tofu, drained spinach, nutmeg, and salt. Set aside. In a small saucepan, melt the butter. Quickly stir in flour and cook for 1 minute. Slowly whisk in the soy milk until mixture is thickened and smooth. Stir sauce into spinach mixture and mix until well combined.

Preheat the oven to 350° F. Spray a 13x9x2-inch glass casserole dish with cooking spray. To assemble the lasagna, place 3 noodles on the bottom of the pan. Spread $1/3$ of the spinach mixture over noodles. Ladle $1/4$ of the sauce (about $1 1/4$ cups) evenly over spinach layer; sprinkle with $1/4$ cup of the Parmesan cheese. Repeat layers twice. Top lasagna with remaining 3 noodles, remaining sauce, and the rest of the Parmesan cheese.

Cover with foil. Bake 40 minutes or until hot and bubbly. Remove foil and bake uncovered for 10 minutes more. Let stand 5 minutes before cutting into squares. Garnish with basil leaves and serve.

Greek Pasta with Tomatoes and Beans

6 to 8 SERVINGS

- $1/4$ cup olive oil
- 2 cloves garlic, minced
- 28-ounce can diced tomatoes with liquid
- 15-ounce can cannellini or navy beans, rinsed and
  drained
- 1 tablespoon chopped fresh basil
- 2 teaspoons chopped fresh oregano
- 4 cups fresh baby spinach leaves
- 1 tablespoon drained capers
- 12 ounces farfalle (bow tie) or penne pasta, cooked
  and drained
- $1/2$ cup crumbled feta cheese
- $1/2$ cup grated Romano cheese

In a large sauté pan, heat the olive oil and sauté the garlic until slightly golden. Add the undrained diced tomatoes, the drained beans, basil, and oregano; bring mixture to boiling. Reduce heat and simmer for 5 minutes. Stir in the fresh spinach and cook for 2 minutes until wilted. Stir in the capers.

To serve, in a large bowl toss the bean mixture with the pasta and the cheeses. Serve with a large salad.

Farfalle with No-Cook Fresh Tomato Sauce

7 to 8 SERVINGS

> 20 Roma tomatoes, skinned, seeded and chopped into
>   bite-sized pieces (approximately 5 cups)*
> ½ cup olive oil
> 8 cloves garlic, halved
> 1 cup chopped fresh basil
> ½ cup freshly grated Romano cheese
> ½ cup fresh chopped parsley
> 1 pound farfalle (bow tie) or any-shaped pasta
> Grated Romano cheese for garnish (optional)

In a large nonmetal bowl, combine the tomatoes with the olive oil, garlic, basil, cheese, and parsley. Allow to sit at room temperature for 2 hours. Remove garlic pieces.

Cook pasta in a large pot of boiling salted water according to package directions. Drain well. Ladle the fresh tomato sauce over the pasta. Sprinkle with additional cheese and serve. This dish is great during the summer months when tomatoes are at the height of the season. Serve hot or cold. The sauce is also excellent for bruschetta.

---

*To easily skin and seed tomatoes, cut a small X with a paring knife on the skin of each tomato; then drop into boiling water. Remove after about 1 minute; cool and peel. If peels don't remove easily, return tomatoes to the boiling water for another minute. Halve tomatoes and scoop out the seeds; a grapefruit spoon works well for this.

Fusilli with Smoked Salmon and Caviar

6 to 8 SERVINGS

1 pound fusilli (corkscrew pasta)
1 ½ cups low-fat ricotta cheese
½ cup nonfat milk
4 ounces (½ cup) soft tofu, drained
4 leaves fresh basil, torn, or 1 teaspoon dried basil,
    crushed
1 clove garlic, minced
1 tablespoon olive oil (optional)
8 ounces smoked salmon, cut into bite-sized strips
½ cup finely chopped red onion
½ cup chopped fresh parsley
1 to 2 tablespoons caviar
2 tablespoons lemon juice
Nonfat dairy sour cream, lemon wedges, and chopped
    parsley for garnish

Cook pasta according to package directions. Meanwhile, in a blender container or food processor bowl, combine ricotta cheese, milk, tofu, basil, and garlic. Cover and blend until smooth. Drain pasta, rinse with cool water, and drain again. (If cooking pasta ahead, toss with olive oil.) Turn into a large shallow serving bowl.

Toss pasta with ricotta sauce, then add salmon, onion, parsley, caviar, and lemon juice and toss well. Garnish each serving with a dollop of sour cream, lemon wedges, and chopped parsley.

VEGETABLES

Spaghetti Squash with Fresh Tomato Sauce

6 TO 8 SERVINGS

1 large spaghetti squash
Olive oil

Fresh tomato sauce:
2 tablespoons olive oil
8 scallions, thinly sliced
8 cloves garlic, halved
⅔ cup white wine
24 Roma tomatoes, peeled, seeded, and chopped
    (approximately 5½ cups)*
¼ cup chopped fresh basil
Salt and pepper to taste
Grated Parmesan or Romano cheese

Preheat oven to 350°F. Rinse and dry the squash, then rub the outside of the squash with olive oil. Pierce the squash a few times with a knife. Place on middle rack of oven and bake for 40 to 50 minutes, or until a knife runs easily through the squash.

Meanwhile, in a large sauté pan, heat the olive oil over medium-high heat; sauté the scallions and garlic

*See my recipe for Farfalle with No-Cook Fresh Tomato Sauce on page 135 for instructions on peeling tomatoes.

until golden. Stir in wine and bring mixture to a simmer; reduce heat and simmer until mixture is reduced by half. Stir in the tomatoes and basil; bring to a boil. Reduce heat and simmer, covered, for 30 minutes. If you prefer a smoother sauce, puree the mixture in a food processor or blender. Season to taste with salt and pepper.

When the squash is done, cut it in half. Scoop out the seeds from the center and discard. With the tines of a fork, scrape out the spaghettilike pulp from the squash and spoon it into a shallow baking dish. Pour the tomato sauce over the squash and sprinkle with Parmesan cheese. Bake for 10 minutes, or until the cheese melts. Garnish with basil leaves, if desired.

Crusty Potato Fillets

2 SERVINGS

Cooking spray
3 medium-size red potatoes, unpeeled
Dash of garlic powder
Dash of onion powder
Salt and pepper to taste
1 tablespoon fresh or dried rosemary

Preheat the oven to 400°F. Spray a baking sheet with olive oil (or vegetable oil) cooking spray. Slice the potatoes very thin and lay them overlapping on the baking sheet. You should end up with about four rows. Spray the potato slices generously with olive oil spray.

Sprinkle on the garlic and onion powder, salt, and pepper. Sprinkle rosemary over the top and bake up to 30 minutes, or until the potatoes are golden. This dish is low in calories. You can enjoy your potatoes without feeling guilty.

Bok Choy

3 TO 4 SERVINGS

2 teaspoons olive oil
4 stalks bok choy with leaves, halved lengthwise and
    bias-sliced
2 cloves garlic, minced
⅓ cup water
¼ cup low-sodium soy sauce
1 teaspoon sesame oil

In a medium skillet, heat olive oil over medium-high heat. Sauté bok choy and garlic about 4 minutes, stirring frequently, until vegetables are slightly golden. Add water, soy sauce, and sesame oil. Cover and steam about 10 minutes, or until tender.

Candied Carrots

4 TO 5 SERVINGS

2 tablespoons clarified butter*
2 cups trimmed, peeled baby carrots, or sliced carrots
1 tablespoon brown sugar
1 tablespoon balsamic vinegar

In a skillet heat the clarified butter over a medium flame and stir in carrots and brown sugar. Sauté over medium-low heat about 10 minutes, or just until crisp-tender, stirring frequently. Do not overcook. Stir in vinegar and serve.

*Clarified butter is butter with the milky solids removed. Since it doesn't burn as easily as regular butter, it's great for browning vegetables. To clarify butter, melt butter in a pan without stirring. When butter is completely melted, slowly and carefully pour the clear top liquid into a bowl, leaving the milky residue in the pan. Discard residue.

MAIN DISHES

Mexican Black Bean Burger

4 SERVINGS

⅔ cup dried black beans, or 16-ounce can black beans,
    rinsed and drained
Water for cooking dried beans
½ medium yellow onion, chopped
2 scallions, sliced
1 teaspoon finely chopped jalapeño pepper, or ½
    teaspoon cayenne pepper (optional)
1 egg white
1 cup seasoned bread crumbs
2 tablespoons chopped cilantro
2 tablespoons corn (fresh, canned, drained, or frozen,
    thawed)
Cooking spray
2 teaspoons olive oil or vegetable oil
4 whole wheat buns, split
Salsa and guacamole for garnish

If using the dry beans, combine the beans and 4 cups
water in a saucepan. Bring to boiling; reduce heat.
Simmer 2 minutes. Remove from heat; cover and let
stand one hour. (Or, omit simmering; soak beans in
cold water overnight in a covered pan.) Drain and
rinse the beans and combine in same pan with 4 cups
fresh water. Bring to boiling; reduce heat. Cover and
simmer for 1 to 1½ hours. Drain well.

In a food processor, place the well-drained beans, onion, scallions, jalapeño, egg white, bread crumbs, cilantro, and corn in that order. Process just until mixed; mixture may still be lumpy. Overmixing will result in a mushy texture. If mixture seems very soft, add a few tablespoons more bread crumbs. With your hands, shape the mixture into 4 3½-inch round patties. Cover and refrigerate for one hour.

Spray a large skillet with cooking spray and add the olive oil. Sauté the patties over medium heat about 3 to 4 minutes per side, until browned. Serve each patty on a whole wheat bun, garnished with salsa and guacamole as desired. You can also serve these burgers wrapped up in a large flour tortilla or tucked inside a pita bread round with the salsa and guacamole.

Low-Fat Crepes with Ratatouille Filling

10 SERVINGS

Crepes:

1 tablespoon Butter Buds
1 tablespoon water
2½ cups whole wheat flour
2 to 2⅛ cups nonfat milk
2 egg whites
¼ cup chopped chives
¼ cup chopped parsley
⅛ teaspoon salt

Ratatouille filling:

Cooking spray
2 cups sliced yellow onions
6 cloves garlic, minced
2 zucchinis, chopped
2 yellow squash, chopped
1 red bell pepper, chopped
4 Japanese eggplants, peeled and chopped
1 cup sliced fresh shiitake mushrooms or brown
    mushrooms
1 cup 1-inch cuts of asparagus
1 16-ounce can diced tomatoes with liquid
½ cup water
¼ cup chopped fresh basil
¼ cup chopped fresh parsley
1 teaspoon salt
1 teaspoon dried oregano, crushed

Topping:

¼ cup grated Parmesan or Romano cheese

For the crepe batter, in a small bowl, stir together the Butter Buds and water. In a large bowl, combine the flour, milk, egg whites, Butter Buds mixture, chives, parsley, and salt until well mixed. Refrigerate batter about one hour or until slightly thickened.

Meanwhile, prepare the ratatouille filling. Spray a Dutch oven or medium stockpot with cooking spray. Sauté onions and garlic over medium heat about 3 minutes or until tender. Stir in zucchini, squash, bell pepper, eggplant, mushrooms, and asparagus. Cook over medium-low heat, stirring frequently, for 10 minutes. Stir in the undrained tomatoes, water, and herbs and seasonings. Bring mixture to boiling. Reduce heat and simmer, partially covered, for 1 hour, stirring frequently.

To cook the crepes, spray a nonstick crepe or omelet pan with cooking spray. Heat pan over high heat. Pour 1/4 cup batter into pan and spread batter to cover bottom of pan. (If batter seems very thick, add a couple of tablespoons milk to thin.) Cook crepe until browned on the bottom, then turn and cook 2 minutes more. Transfer each crepe to a warm platter, placing a sheet of paper towel between pancakes. Repeat with remaining crepe batter.

To assemble crepes, preheat oven to 350°F. Spray a 12 × 8 × 2-inch baking dish with cooking spray. Spoon about 1/3 cup of the vegetable mixture over each crepe, roll up, and place seam-side down in baking dish. Spoon any remaining vegetable mixture over top of crepes. Sprinkle with cheese. Cover with foil and bake for 20 minutes or until heated through.

Thai Sweet-and-Sour Prawns

4 SERVINGS

1/4 cup water
3 tablespoons catsup
1 1/2 tablespoons Thai fish sauce*
1 tablespoon lemon juice
1 tablespoon oyster sauce
1 tablespoon natural sugar
2 tablespoons peanut oil or olive oil
3 cloves garlic, minced
1 cup fresh pineapple chunks
1 large diced tomato
1 peeled and cubed cucumber
1 pound large prawns, peeled and deveined, or 12 ounces
    (1 1/2 cups) extra-firm tofu, cut into bite-size pieces
1/2 cup chopped scallions
Hot cooked Thai noodles, rice noodles, or rice
Chopped cilantro for garnish (optional)

In a bowl stir together the water, catsup, fish sauce, lemon juice, oyster sauce, and sugar until well blended. Set aside. In a large wok or skillet, heat the oil until very hot. Add the garlic and stir-fry 1 minute. Add the pineapple, tomato, and cucumber; stir-fry for 2 minutes. Stir the fish sauce mixture; add to the wok. Bring mixture to simmering and add the prawns. Simmer over low heat, stirring frequently until prawns turn pink and opaque. (If you choose to use tofu, heat until tofu is browned.)

Stir in the scallions. Serve mixture on a platter with Thai noodles, rice noodles, or rice. Garnish with chopped cilantro, if desired.

*Thai fish sauce can be found in larger supermarkets or in specialty or Asian food markets.

Oriental Roasted Salmon

4 SERVINGS

1-pound salmon fillet, cut into 4 pieces
Cooking spray
1/3 cup Dijon mustard
2 tablespoons soy sauce
1 tablespoon mirin (sweet rice wine)
1 tablespoon grated fresh gingerroot
1 teaspoon sesame oil
1 to 3 teaspoons cracked pepper (optional)
4 scallions, trimmed
1/2 red bell pepper, cut into julienne strips
1/2 green bell pepper, cut into julienne strips
Lemon and lime wedges for garnish

Preheat broiler. Place the salmon pieces on a nonstick broiler pan sprayed with cooking spray. In a small bowl, combine the mustard, soy sauce, mirin, gingerroot, oil, and pepper (if desired). Spread half of the mixture over the fish. Cut scallions in half crosswise, then lengthwise into long, thin strips. Set aside. Broil salmon 4 inches from the heat for 3 minutes. Turn salmon pieces with tongs; brush remaining mustard mixture over fish. Broil 2 minutes more. Spoon the scallions and bell peppers evenly over fish pieces. Broil 2 to 3 minutes more, or until vegetables are slightly charred and fish flakes easily with a fork. Serve immediately with lemon and lime wedges. Serve with sticky rice and Bok Choy (see page 140) for a lovely light dinner or lunch.

Sea Bass with Lemon and Capers

4 SERVINGS

 1 cup all-purpose flour
 1 teaspoon salt
 ½ teaspoon pepper
 1-pound sea bass, cut into 4 pieces
 Cooking spray
 1 tablespoon olive oil
 4 cloves garlic, sliced
 ½ cup dry white wine
 ⅓ cup fresh lemon juice
 2 tablespoons soy sauce
 ½ cup chopped Italian parsley
 2 tablespoons drained capers
 Italian parsley and thinly sliced lemons for garnish
    (optional)

In a shallow bowl stir together the flour, salt, and pepper. Coat sea bass on all sides with flour mixture; set aside.

Spray a large skillet with cooking spray; add oil. Sauté the sea bass with the garlic over medium-high heat for about 5 to 6 minutes, turning after 3 minutes to brown evenly. Add wine, lemon juice, and soy sauce. Cover and simmer for 2 minutes. Stir in parsley and capers. Serve immediately, garnished with Italian parsley and sliced lemons, if desired. Serve with Candied Carrots (page 141) and steamed broccoli with olive oil, lemon, salt, and pepper.

Raspberry-Glazed Chicken

4 SERVINGS

> 1/2 cup all-purpose flour
> 1 teaspoon dried thyme, crushed
> 1/4 teaspoon salt
> 4 boned, skinned chicken breasts
> 3 tablespoons olive oil
> 1 cup chopped red onion
> 1/4 cup white wine
> 1/2 cup raspberry preserves
> 2 tablespoons balsamic vinegar
> Hot cooked rice or steamed greens

In a shallow bowl, stir together flour, thyme, and salt. Coat the chicken breasts on all sides in the flour mixture. Set aside.

In a large sauté pan, heat the olive oil. Sauté the red onion over low heat until tender, about 5 minutes. Add the chicken breasts and sauté for 5 to 6 minutes per side until golden brown and no longer pink in the center.

Remove the chicken to a warm platter; cover and keep warm. Add the wine to the pan, scraping up any crusty bits on the bottom of the pan; simmer until mixture is reduced by half. Stir in the preserves and the vinegar; cook a few minutes more until preserves are melted.

To serve, spoon the sauce over the chicken, and serve with hot cooked rice or steamed greens.

Cornmeal-Crusted Chicken

8 SERVINGS

2 pounds skinned chicken pieces, or chicken breasts
1 cup low-fat buttermilk
1/2 cup yellow cornmeal
1/2 cup seasoned bread crumbs
1/2 cup grated Parmesan cheese
1 teaspoon salt
1/2 teaspoon pepper
1 egg plus one egg white
Butter-flavored cooking spray

Remove excess fat from chicken pieces. Coat chicken on all sides with the buttermilk. Cover and refrigerate for 30 minutes.

Preheat oven to 425°F. In a shallow bowl, stir together the cornmeal, bread crumbs, Parmesan cheese, salt, and pepper. In another shallow bowl whisk together the egg and egg white until frothy. Dip the chicken pieces first into the beaten eggs, then coat thoroughly with the cornmeal mixture. Place the coated pieces on a rack, set onto a baking sheet. Spray the chicken lightly with butter-flavored cooking spray.

Bake uncovered for 35 to 45 minutes, or until golden brown and no longer pink in the center.

Thai Minced Chicken in Lettuce Leaves

5 TO 6 SERVINGS

    3 tablespoons Thai fish sauce*
    2 tablespoons lemon juice
    1/2 teaspoon crushed red pepper flakes
    1 tablespoon arrowroot or cornstarch
    1/3 cup soy sauce
    1 tablespoon peanut oil or olive oil
    1 medium onion, cut into bite-size pieces
    4 scallions, sliced
    3 tablespoons grated fresh gingerroot
    2 cloves garlic, minced
    5 boned, skinned chicken breasts, chopped
    2 tablespoons chopped peanuts
    2 tablespoons chopped cilantro
    1 tablespoon chopped fresh mint
    5 to 6 large leaves iceberg or romaine lettuce

In a small bowl stir together the fish sauce, lemon juice, and red pepper flakes. Set aside. In another small bowl stir arrowroot or cornstarch into soy sauce until dissolved. Set aside.

In a wok or large skillet heat the oil until very hot. Stir-fry the onion, scallions, gingerroot, and garlic for 2 minutes. Add the chicken and stir-fry for about 4 minutes, or until meat is no longer pink. Stir in the fish sauce mixture and cook 1 minute more.

Push the meat mixture to the sides of the wok. Stir the soy sauce mixture again; add it to the center of the wok and cook and stir until thickened and bub-

*Thai fish sauce can be found in larger supermarkets or in specialty or Asian food markets.

bly. Cook 1 minute more. Stir in the peanuts, cilantro, and mint.

To serve, spoon some of the mixture onto a lettuce leaf and roll up like a burrito.

Good-for-You Cheeseburgers with Unfried Potatoes

4 SERVINGS

2 stalks celery, chopped
1 1/2 pounds ground white turkey meat
1 tablespoon Spike salt-free seasoning
1/4 cup plain bread crumbs
1/2 cup chopped scallions
Cooking spray
1 tablespoon olive oil or vegetable oil
1/2 cup soy sauce
1/2 cup nonfat or lowfat mayonnaise
3 tablespoons catsup
1 tablespoon pickle relish
1 teaspoon bottled hot pepper sauce (optional)
4 1-ounce slices low-fat cheese
4 whole wheat buns, split, and warmed if desired

Cook celery in a small amount of boiling water until tender; drain well. In a large bowl, combine the turkey, seasoning, bread crumbs, cooked celery, and scallions. Shape mixture with hands into 4 patties.

Spray a large, nonstick skillet with cooking spray and add oil; heat until hot. Cook burger patties over medium-high heat for 3 minutes. Turn and cook 3 minutes more. Add the soy sauce and reduce heat. Cover and simmer for 2 to 3 minutes or until patties are no longer pink in the center.

Meanwhile, prepare sauce: In a small bowl stir together the mayonnaise, catsup, relish, and pepper sauce (if desired). Place one slice cheese on each patty; cover and remove from heat. Let stand 1 to 2 minutes until cheese melts. Serve each patty on a bun topped with some of the sauce. (For heated buns, wrap them in foil and heat in a 350°F oven for 15 minutes. Or, toast them if you desire.)

Unfried Potatoes
4 large Idaho potatoes, cut into sticks
2 large egg whites, beaten until frothy
1 tablespoon Cajun seasoning or Spike seasoning
Cooking spray

Preheat oven to 400°F. In a large bowl, toss together the sliced potatoes with the egg whites and seasoning. Spray a baking sheet with cooking spray and arrange potatoes on baking sheet. Bake for 35 to 40 minutes, turning often until fries are crisp and golden. Serve with burgers.

ANYTIME SNACKS AND SMOOTHIES

Soybean Hummus

3 CUPS

1 cup dry soybeans, or 2 15-ounce cans soybeans,
   rinsed and drained
1/4 cup olive oil
1/4 cup lemon juice
1 tablespoon balsamic vinegar
1 tablespoon Dijon mustard
4 sprigs parsley
2 cloves garlic, quartered
1/4 teaspoon salt
1/4 teaspoon pepper
Pita bread triangles

If using dry soybeans, combine the beans and 8 cups water in a Dutch oven or stockpot. Bring to boiling; reduce heat. Simmer for 2 minutes. Remove from heat; cover and let stand 1 hour. (Or, omit simmering; soak beans in cold water overnight in a covered pan.) Drain and rinse the beans and combine in same pan with 8 cups fresh water. Bring to boiling; reduce heat. Cover and simmer for 2 to 2½ hours. Drain well.

In a blender or food processor, combine beans, oil, lemon juice, vinegar, mustard, parsley, garlic, salt, and pepper. Cover and blend until smooth. Serve with toasted pita bread cut into triangles.

I serve this to my kids as a healthy snack. They use it as a dip with not only pita bread but celery or carrot sticks, salt-free pretzels, toast, and rice cakes.

Low-Fat Egg Rolls

20 EGG ROLLS

8 dried shiitake mushrooms
Cooking spray
1 tablespoon olive oil or vegetable oil
2 cups julienne-cut carrots
3 stalks celery, thinly sliced
1 cup bean sprouts
1 cup snow peas, stringed and sliced lengthwise
2 teaspoons grated fresh gingerroot
4 cloves garlic, minced
1/2 cup cooked diced chicken, shrimp, or a combination
4 ounces (1/2 cup) extra-firm tofu, drained and cut into
    bite-size pieces
1 teaspoon arrowroot or cornstarch
20 egg roll wrappers

Dipping sauce:
3/4 cup low-sodium soy sauce
1/4 cup seasoned rice-wine vinegar
1 tablespoon toasted sesame seeds*
1/2 teaspoon red pepper flakes (optional)

Hot mustard sauce:
2 tablespoons catsup
1 teaspoon Chinese mustard or hot mustard

Place mushrooms in a small saucepan with water to
cover. Bring to boiling; boil 2 minutes. Remove from

---

*To toast the sesame seeds, simply place in a nonstick frying pan and
sauté over the stove until they turn golden brown. Take care not to burn
them. You can also toast sesame seeds on the top brown setting in a
toaster oven, but watch them carefully. Sesame seeds have a rich, full-
bodied flavor when toasted.

heat; let stand 5 minutes. Remove mushrooms, re-
serving liquid. Drain well and slice.

Spray a wok or large skillet with cooking spray.
Add oil; heat until very hot. Sauté carrots, celery, the
sliced mushrooms, bean sprouts, snow peas, gingerroot, and garlic, stir-frying for 3 to 5 minutes, or until
vegetables are crisp-tender. (If vegetables begin to
stick to the pan, add a tablespoon or two of the reserved mushroom-soaking liquid.) Stir in chicken
and/or shrimp and the tofu.

In a small bowl stir together 2 teaspoons of the
reserved mushroom liquid and arrowroot until dissolved. Add to wok; cook and stir 1 minute. Remove
from heat; allow mixture to cool slightly.

Spray a large baking sheet with cooking spray. To
assemble each egg roll, place an egg roll wrapper on
a flat surface with one point facing you. Spoon ⅛ cup
of the filling mixture across the center of the egg roll
skin. Fold bottom point of skin over filling, and tuck
point under filling. Moisten the side corners with
water, then fold them over, forming an envelope
shape. Roll up egg roll toward top corner, then
moisten point with water and press down firmly to
seal. Repeat to make about 20 egg rolls.

Place egg rolls side by side, about ¼ inch apart, on
the baking sheet. Cover and refrigerate for 1 hour.
Preheat oven to 400° F. Bake for 20 to 25 minutes or
until light golden brown, turning rolls once with
tongs after about 15 minutes to brown both sides
evenly.

These egg rolls are amazingly good baked. However, they can be fried the traditional way in a wok
with a couple inches of olive or peanut oil heated to
365° F. Fry 2 to 3 minutes or until golden brown. Ob-

viously, when fried these eggrolls will not be low-fat, but now and again frying won't hurt you. Let them cool slightly before serving.

Meanwhile, combine ingredients for dipping sauce and hot mustard sauce. Cool slightly and serve egg rolls whole or halved (cut on the diagonal) with sauces.

Snack Foods

My biggest downfall is snacks—the crunchy, salty ones. I love 'em! Potato chips, peanuts, and cheese-flavored snacks are hard for me to resist. I had to come up with some healthy alternatives to my cravings, to avoid going back to my old way of munching. Here are the snacks that work for me. As long as I stick to these, I have no problems sticking to my program. Let me share them with you:

Rice cakes

My favorite ones are the popcorn-flavored rice cakes, and I also enjoy the plain brown rice cakes.

SUGGESTED TOPPINGS FOR RICE CAKES

- 2 tablespoons Caraway Tuna Salad (page 129)
- 1 tablespoon reduced-fat peanut butter
- 1 tablespoon Soybean Hummus (page 155) or regular hummus
- 2 tablespoons Terrific Tofu "Egg" Salad (page 127), or regular egg salad
- 2 teaspoons desired flavor fruit preserves (my personal favorite is cherry)

Pretzels

I prefer them unsalted. You can dip them in hummus and low-fat peanut butter, or enjoy them plain. Pretzels are low in fat.

Bagels

I hollow out ½ bagel, toast it, and spread it with a little tuna, or nonfat or low-fat cream cheese. You can also sprinkle it with 2 tablespoons shredded low-fat cheese and run it under the broiler to melt the cheese.

Nonfat yogurt

I recommend any flavor. One of my favorite snacks involves heaping 2 tablespoons of vanilla-flavored yogurt over one cut-up apple, then sprinkling the whole thing with ground cinnamon, raisins, and 3 crushed almonds. It's a great pick-me-up.

Fruit-flavored soy drinks

Look for them in the dairy case at your supermarket or health food store. A serving is 6 ounces.

Strawberry or Raspberry Puree

I make my own quick Strawberry or Raspberry Puree: Place in the blender 2 cups washed and hulled strawberries or raspberries, 1 cup orange juice, and 2 tablespoons sugar. Puree, then strain to remove seeds. Pour this sauce over fresh berries, nonfat frozen yogurt, or sorbet. It keeps for one week in the refrigerator.

Angel food cake

Another food that contains little fat; you can buy these in the supermarket or make one yourself, from a mix or from scratch. Serve yourself a slice with fresh berry slices and a spoonful of raspberry or strawberry glaze.

Crudites

Help yourself to any kind of fresh raw vegetable and dip into a yogurt dip or balsamic vinaigrette. Or try:

Celery Rings

1 cup minced cooked chicken
2 tablespoons nonfat cream cheese
1 tablespoon lemon juice
1 tablespoon nonfat mayonnaise
1 scallion, thinly sliced, or 1 tablespoon chopped
   chives
2 drops bottled hot pepper sauce (optional)
Celery stalks with leaves

In a food processor or blender, combine first 6 ingredients until well blended. Spoon into celery stalks. Top with another celery stalk, upside down, to make a cylinder shape. Slice crosswise into ½-inch pieces. You can also use just the cream cheese and omit the chicken.

Bran Muffin

I heat one and serve it with a 6-ounce glass of ice-cold nonfat milk. See the recipe on page 101.

Soy Nuts

Toast them in a toaster oven. About ½ cup is a serving.

Soy Pods

I like to steam them; again, ½ cup is a serving.

Miso soup

See the recipe on page 117.

Strawberry-Banana Tofu Smoothie

2 TO 3 SERVINGS

½ cup apple juice
½ cup frozen vanilla nonfat yogurt, peach sorbet, or
    desired flavor sorbet
4 ounces (½ cup) soft tofu, drained
1 cup fresh or frozen sliced strawberries or peaches
1 banana, broken into chunks
1 teaspoon honey
½ cup ice cubes
Fresh whole berries for garnish (optional)

In a blender container, place the apple juice, sorbet, tofu, strawberries or peaches, banana, and honey. Cover and process until smooth. Through hole in lid of blender, with machine running, add ice cubes one at a time until smooth and well-blended. Pour into tall glasses; garnish with a fresh berry, if desired.

Orange Velvet Deluxe

3 TO 4 SERVINGS

⅔ cup fresh grapefruit juice
⅓ cup fresh orange juice
4 ounces (½ cup) soft tofu, drained
½ cup orange or peach sherbet or sorbet
2 bananas, broken into chunks
1 cup fresh or frozen halved strawberries
1 cup ice cubes
Fresh mint leaves for garnish (optional)

In a blender container, place the juices, tofu, sherbet or sorbet, bananas, and berries. Cover and blend until smooth. Through hole in lid of blender, with machine running, add ice cubes one at a time until smooth and well-blended. Pour into tall glasses; garnish with fresh mint, if desired.

Banana-Chocolate Soyprise

2 SERVINGS

1 cup nonfat or low-fat chocolate soy milk
$\frac{1}{2}$ cup chocolate or vanilla frozen yogurt
2 ounces ($\frac{1}{4}$ cup) soft tofu, drained
2 bananas, broken into chunks
1 tablespoon chocolate syrup
$\frac{1}{2}$ cup ice cubes

In a blender container place the milk, yogurt, tofu, banana chunks, and chocolate syrup. Cover and blend until smooth. Through hole in lid of blender, with machine running, add ice cubes one at a time until smooth and well-blended. Pour into tall glasses.

Perfect Piña Colada
(Alcohol-free)

3 TO 4 SERVINGS

    1 cup pineapple juice
    1 cup fresh pineapple chunks
    1/2 cup vanilla frozen yogurt
    2 ounces (1/4 cup) soft tofu
    1 teaspoon rum extract
    1 teaspoon coconut extract
    1 cup ice cubes
    Fresh mint sprigs for garnish (optional)

In a blender container combine the pineapple juice, pineapple chunks, yogurt, tofu, and extracts. Cover and blend until smooth. Through hole in lid of blender, add ice cubes one at a time until smooth and well-blended. Pour into long-stemmed goblets. Garnish with mint sprigs if desired.

Strawberry Soup

4 SERVINGS

2 pint baskets of fresh strawberries, washed, hulled,
    and cut in half
2 cups of freshly squeezed orange juice
Fresh mint for garnish

Split the strawberries among 4 bowls. Pour the orange juice over the strawberries, then garnish with fresh mint. Serve cold.

I serve Strawberry Soup for breakfast and as a snack. It's a great pick-me-up, and so good for you! Or, you can serve it over angel food cake. Top with nonfat whipped cream.

DESSERTS

Banana Split

1 banana, peeled and split lengthwise
1 scoop nonfat frozen yogurt
6 strawberries, cut into bite-size pieces
1/4 cup blueberries
1/4 cup fresh pineapple chunks
2 tablespoons Strawberry Sauce (see recipe below)
1 teaspoon chocolate syrup

Place the banana in a serving dish. Add the frozen yogurt. Spoon all the fresh fruit on top. Drizzle on the Strawberry Sauce and chocolate syrup.

Strawberry Sauce:
1 pint fresh strawberries, washed and hulled
1 cup fresh orange juice
1 tablespoon sugar

Place all ingredients in blender and blend until smooth. Strain through a sieve to remove the tiny seeds. Store in a glass container. Sauce will last for about five days in the refrigerator. You can use this sauce on many different desserts, especially fruit and even cake.

Soy-Enriched Creamy Rice Pudding

3 TO 4 SERVINGS

1 ⅓ cups vanilla-flavored soy milk
2 cups nonfat milk
⅔ cup Arborio rice or short-grain rice
½ cup natural sugar
¼ teaspoon salt
½ cup raisins
¼ cup golden raisins
3 tablespoons pure maple syrup
1 teaspoon vanilla extract
2 teaspoons cinnamon
Dash nutmeg

Over medium heat in a heavy saucepan, combine the soy milk, milk, rice, sugar, salt, and raisins. Bring to a boil and stir once or twice. Reduce the heat and simmer gently for about 30 to 40 minutes, or until the rice is tender and the mixture is thick.

Add the syrup and vanilla. Mix thoroughly and pour into glass dishes. Sprinkle the cinnamon and nutmeg on top.

Serve warm, or cover with plastic wrap and refrigerate until chilled.

Apple Phyllo

9 SERVINGS

- ¼ cup bread crumbs
- ¼ cup firmly packed brown sugar
- ½ cup granulated sugar
- ¼ teaspoon nutmeg
- ½ teaspoon cinnamon
- ¼ cup raisins
- 4 green apples, peeled, skinned and chopped into pieces
- ½ cup chopped walnuts (optional)
- 1 tablespoon lemon zest
- 1 tablespoon unbleached flour
- 9 sheets phyllo dough, thawed
- Butter-flavored cooking spray

Preheat oven to 350° F. Combine bread crumbs and brown sugar in a bowl. Set aside.

In another bowl combine the sugar, nutmeg, cinnamon, raisins, apples, nuts, lemon zest, and flour. Set aside.

Spray one phyllo sheet lightly with the vegetable spray. (Remember to cover the remaining phyllo sheets with a kitchen towel to keep them from drying out.) Place another sheet on top of that one and spray again. Repeat with the third sheet of phyllo, forming a stack of three sheets. Sprinkle about 2 tablespoons of the bread crumb and sugar mixture on top of the stack.

Using a sharp knife, cut the stack lengthwise into 3 4½-inch-wide strips. Spoon ⅓ cup of the apple mixture onto one end of each strip.

For each strip, fold the left bottom corner over

apple mixture, forming a triangle. Fold that triangle up onto the strip, and keep folding to the end of the strip, as you would fold a flag. Repeat with remaining sheets of phyllo.

Place triangles seam-side down on a baking sheet coated with cooking spray. Bake for 25 minutes, or until golden. Serve with frozen vanilla yogurt or low-fat vanilla ice cream.

Peach Phyllo Dessert Cups

6 SERVINGS

> 6 ripe peaches, peeled and sliced
> 1 teaspoon lemon juice
> 1 tablespoon flour
> 1 teaspoon cinnamon, plus extra for sprinkling
> 1 tablespoon brown or natural sugar, plus extra for
> sprinkling
> 6 sheets phyllo dough
> Butter-flavored cooking spray

Preheat oven to 350° F. Place the peaches in a glass bowl and mix in the lemon juice. Add flour, cinnamon, and sugar. Mix and set aside.

Take one sheet of phyllo and place on cutting board. Cut into twelve squares.

Place one square into the muffin pan and gently press down to form a cup. Spray with butter-flavored spray.

Sprinkle a little sugar and cinnamon in between layers. Add second layer and continue until you have used up all twelve sheets. Add two heaping tablespoons of the peach mixture.

Place in oven and bake for 20 minutes or until the phyllo is a golden, flaky brown. Serve warm right out of the oven with a generous helping of vanilla yogurt, or cool.

Other uses for phyllo cups

Bake your phyllo cups separately and fill with all kinds of yummy things!

• Place your favorite sorbet inside a baked cup. Mine is peach. I serve it with a raspberry glaze and drizzle on some chocolate sauce. I also add a few berries on top. It makes a wonderfully refreshing dessert.

• Mix fresh berries such as strawberries, raspberries, and blueberries.

Place all the berries in a bowl, add ½ cup fresh orange juice, and mix. Drop a dollop of whipped cream on the bottom of a baked cup (a dollop never hurt anyone!), add the fresh berries, then garnish with a chopped leaf of fresh mint.

• Place two heaping tablespoons of your favorite cherry pie filling into each cup and bake.

• Drop a scoop of frozen yogurt into each cup, and top with some combination of fresh fruit, raspberry glaze, and chocolate sauce.

Raspberry or strawberry glaze:
2 pints raspberries or strawberries, cleaned and
    hulled
Juice of 2 oranges
1 teaspoon arrowroot
2 tablespoons sugar

Place raspberries or strawberries in a blender. Add the juice, arrowroot, and sugar. Blend and strain through a sieve to remove the tiny seeds. The glaze will keep for 3 days if refrigerated in a glass jar.

Chocolate Brownies

6 TO 8 SERVINGS

Whenever I have an urge for chocolate I eat these. At least they are low in fat and calories—approximately 120 calories and 1 gram of fat!

Cooking spray
3/4 cup unbleached flour
1/2 cup cocoa powder
1 teaspoon baking powder
1/2 teaspoon baking soda
1 large banana
1/2 cup unsweetened apple juice
3/4 cup light brown sugar
1 1/2 teaspoon vanilla extract
1 tablespoon instant espresso coffee granules
1/3 cup chopped walnuts (optional)
4 large egg whites
1/2 teaspoon salt

Preheat oven to 350° F. Spray an 8x8-inch baking pan with cooking spray.

In a bowl combine flour, cocoa powder, baking powder, and baking soda.

In a food processor with a mixer, blend banana, apple juice, brown sugar, vanilla, espresso granules, and salt until smooth. Fold in walnuts.

Beat the egg whites with the salt until soft peaks form. Fold half the egg whites into the batter. Mix gently. Add the remaining egg whites and mix gently.

Pour into the pan and spread evenly. Bake for 30 to 35 minutes, or until the brownie pops back when pushed gently in the center. Cool in the pan. Cut into squares, and serve with nonfat fudge sauce on top.

BIBLIOGRAPHY

These are the books that I relied on when researching for this book. You may want to consult them for further information.

Castleman, Michael and Sheldon Saul Hendler. *The Healing Herbs: The Ultimate Guide to the Curative Power of Nature's Medicines.* New York: Bantam Books, 1995.

Dorland, W. A. Newman. *Dorland's Illustrated Medical Dictionary.* 28th Ed. Philadelphia: W.B. Saunders Co., 1994.

Editors of Time Life Books. *The Medical Advisor: The Complete Guide to Alternative and Conventional Treatments.* New York: Time Life Books, 1996.

Hadady, Letha, D. AC. *Asian Health Secrets: The Complete Guide to Asian Herbal Medicine.* New York: Three Rivers Press, 1998.

Heinerman, John. *Heinerman's Encyclopedia of Healing Herbs and Spices.* Paramus, N.J.: Prentice Hall Trade, 1996.

Huston, James E., M.D. and L. Darlene Lanka, M.D. *Perimenopause.* Oakland, Calif.: New Harbinger Publications, Inc., 1997.

Love, Susan, M.D. with Karen Lindsay. *Dr. Susan Love's Hormone Book: Making Informed Choices*

About Menopause. New York: Random House, 1998.

Martin, Raquel with Judi Gerstrung. *The Estrogen Alternative: Natural Hormone Therapy with Botanical Progesterone.* Rochester, N.Y.: Healing Arts Press, 1998.

Murray, Michael T. *Encyclopedia of Nutritional Supplements: The Essential Guide for Improving Your Health Naturally.* Rocklin, Calif.: Prima Publishing, 1996.

Northrup, Christiane, M.D. *Women's Bodies, Women's Wisdom: Creating Physical and Emotional Health and Healing.* New York: Bantam Doubleday Dell Publishing Group, Inc., 1998.

Pitchford, Paul. *Healing with Whole Foods: Oriental Traditions and Modern Nutrition.* 2nd ed. Berkeley: North Atlantic Books, 1996.

Pressman, Alan H., Sheila Buff, and Gary Null. *The Complete Idiot's Guide to Vitamins and Minerals.* Malibu, Calif.: Alpha Books, 1998.

Reichman, Judith, M.D. *I'm Not in the Mood: What Every Woman Should Know About Improving Her Libido.* New York: William Morrow & Co., 1998.

————. *I'm Too Young to Get Old: Health Care for Women over Forty.* New York: Times Books, 1997.

Rosenfeld, Isadore, M.D. *Doctor, What Should I Eat? Nutrition Prescriptions for Ailments in Which Diet Can Really Make a Difference.* New York: Warner Books, 1996.

Shandler, Nina. *Estrogen: The Natural Way: Over 250*

Easy and Delicious Recipes for Menopause. New York: Villard Books, 1997.

Weil, Andrew, M.D. *8 Weeks to Optimum Health: A Proven Program for Taking Full Advantage of Your Body's Natural Healing Power.* New York: Knopf, 1997.